# THE 36-HOUR DAY

Nancy L. Mace and
Peter V. Rabins, M.D.

A Family Guide to Caring for Persons with Alzheimer's Disease, Related Dementing Illnesses, and Memory Loss in Later Life

0-446-32201-6 $3.95 (U.S.A.)

ISBN 0-446-32201-6

"*The 36-Hour Day* is a gift for families who struggle with the frustrations involved in caring for a loved one stricken by dementing illness. It's a practical book, perhaps even more important for its message to those families. That message is: 'You are not alone.'"
—Congressman Claude Pepper, Chairman,
House Select Committee on Aging

"Excellent guidance and clear information of a kind that the family needs when facing such a tragedy."
—Harold M. Schmeck, Jr.,
*The New York Times*

"Meticulous, practical, and sympathetic...Superb guidance and support for families faced with a devastating problem."

—*Kirkus Reviews*

"A very useful book...It offers a wealth of knowledge on how to cope with the impaired family member. *The 36-Hour Day* is the best available guide on this subject."
—William Reichel, M.D., Chairman,
Board of Directors,
American Geriatrics Society

NANCY L. MACE is assistant in psychiatry and coordinator of the T. Rowe and Eleanor Price Teaching Service in the Department of Psychiatry at The Johns Hopkins University School of Medicine.

PETER V. RABINS, M.D., a geriatric psychiatrist, is director of the Price Teaching Service and assistant professor of psychiatry at The Johns Hopkins University School of Medicine.

**Endorsed by the Alzheimer's Disease and Related Disorders Association of America**

# THE 36-HOUR DAY

A Family Guide to Caring for
Persons with Alzheimer's Disease,
Related Dementing Illnesses,
and Memory Loss in Later Life

NANCY L. MACE
PETER V. RABINS, M.D.

WARNER BOOKS

A Warner Communications Company

WARNER BOOKS EDITION

**Copyright © 1981** *by The Johns Hopkins University Press.*
**All rights reserved.**

This Warner Books Edition is published by arrangement with
*The Johns Hopkins University Press,*
*Baltimore, Maryland 21218*

*Warner Books, Inc.,*
*666 Fifth Avenue,*
*New York, N.Y. 10103*

A Warner Communications Company

*Printed in the United States of America*

**First Warner Books Printing:** *April, 1984*

**10 9 8 7 6 5 4 3 2 1**

This book is dedicated to
*everyone who gives a "36-hour-day"*
*to the care of a person with a dementing illness.*

# CONTENTS

vii

## Contents

viii

# Contents

## Contents

# Contents

# Contents

## Contents

# THE 36-HOUR DAY

# FOREWORD

The need for a practical and detailed reference book to assist family members of patients with dementia has long been felt. Many of these families would be prepared to continue caring for their relatives at home if they understood some issues better and in that way could manage their problems better. A more complete understanding of the nature of the symptoms and some of the troublesome behaviors that occasionally accompany these conditions would make the disorders seem much less mysterious and the implications of symptoms much less threatening.

In fact, the symptoms and accompanying troubles of demented patients are much more straightforward than those of many other patients with psychiatric disorders. And yet, patients suffering from these various dementing illnesses have not been described, nor have their families been helped. This deficiency, the result of longstanding neglect of issues affecting the elderly, is now being corrected by initiatives such as this one. The sense of pessimism and helplessness that has characterized the care of these patients in the past is being replaced by a new optimism derived from a special concern for patients' well-being. The likely outcome is not only better care for these patients but also an interest in their management that will manifest itself in research and teaching. This book represents the first step in these directions and can be read either as a means of providing immediate direction on pressing problems or as an overall approach to the care and treatment of the patient throughout the course of his or her dementing condition.

*The 36-Hour Day* is a tribute to the far-thinking people who began a program directed at the needs of people with dementing illnesses at The Hopkins Medical Institutions, including the authors, and to the T. Rowe and Eleanor Price Foundation, which supported this program. Philanthropy used to enhance care giving and provide instruction on particular care-giving methods is rather rare, but it is especially needed in this area.

Paul R. McHugh, M.D.
*Director and Psychiatrist in Chief*
*Department of Psychiatry and Behavioral Sciences*
*The Johns Hopkins University School of Medicine*

Although this book was written for the families of people with dementing illnesses, we recognize that other people, including those suffering from these conditions, may read this book. We welcome this. We hope that the use of such words as *patient* and *brain-injured person* will not discourage those who have these illnesses. These words were chosen because we want to emphasize that the people who suffer from these conditions are ill, not ''just old.'' We hope the tone of the book conveys that we think of you as individuals and people and never as objects.

This book is not intended to provide medical or legal advice. The services of a competent professional should be obtained when legal, medical, or other specific advice is needed.

At present, not all professionals are knowledgeable about dementia. We frequently refer to trained personnel who can help you, but we recognize that you may have difficulty finding the help you need. You, the care giver, will need to utilize both professional resources and your own good judgment. This book cannot address the particulars of your situation, but is intended only as a general guide.

In addition, we recognize that often resources such as day care, in-home care, or evaluation programs are not available or their availability may change, and that many such resources are dependent on federal funds and therefore on federal policy.

We use examples of family situations to illustrate our discussion. These examples are not descriptions of real families or patients. They are based upon experiences, feelings, and solutions that families and patients have discussed with us. Names and other identifying information have been changed.

Both men and women suffer from these diseases. To simplify reading, we will use the masculine pronouns *he* and *his* and the feminine pronouns *she* and *hers* in alternate chapters.

# ACKNOWLEDGMENTS

So many people have given of their time, experience, and wisdom that it is not possible to name them all. We wish to thank all those known and anonymous who have contributed ideas and information.

The T. Rowe and Eleanor Price Foundation, through the establishment of the T. Rowe and Eleanor Price Teaching Service in the Department of Psychiatry and Behavioral Sciences at The Johns Hopkins University School of Medicine, has brought together a team of people to learn about and teach the care of persons with a dementing illness. Paul R. McHugh, M.D., director and psychiatrist in chief of the Department of Psychiatry and Behavioral Sciences, has made the study of the dementias and their impact on families and patients a major focus of the department. Many of the ideas presented here are his. He has also read the entire manuscript, contributed to its form and content, and advised us throughout its development. Marshal F. Folstein, M.D., director of the Division of General Hospital Psychiatry, has taught us much about the care of patients and their families and has been a source of many of the ideas presented in this book. Ernest M. Gruenberg, M.D., Ph.D., and Morton Kramer, Sc.D., have added to our understanding of the social impact of dementia.

Our colleagues have made significant contributions to the content of the book. Jeanne M. Floyd, R.N., developed many of the management techniques we discuss and has worked closely with us in making specific suggestions about care. Together with the nursing staff of the psychogeriatric unit of the Phipps Clinic and Head Nurse Eva Ridder, R.N., she has developed and tested many new ideas. Janet Abrams Bachur, A.C.S.W., wrote sections of the material on finding resources and selecting a nursing home. She also read much of the manuscript and contributed to it her extensive knowledge of resources and family therapy. Sue R. Hardy, O.T.R., has researched, developed, and tested much of the material on occupational and physical therapy. Jeanne, Janet, and Sue helped compile the reading list.

Mary Jane Lucas, R.N., shared with us her extensive knowledge of patients and families who suffer from these illnesses. Her group therapy with spouses of patients suffering from dementia has shaped our general knowledge of families' emotional reactions and our specific ideas about group work with family members. Jerome D. Frank, M.D., Ph.D., read and commented on the section of the manuscript which discusses emotions.

Most important among those who have taught us are our patients and their families. From them we have learned of problems, solutions, and, most important, the strength, courage, and love with which families and patients face the dementing illnesses. Many members of the Alzheimer's Disease Association of Maryland (ADAM) and the Alzheimer's Disease and Related Disorders Association (ADRDA) have read the manuscript, contributed to it, and taken the time to call, write, and share solutions to problems they have faced. It is not possible to name each of them, but we especially wish to thank Glenn I. Kirkland, Mary LaRue, Bobbie Glaze, John J. Mitchell, Joan and Douglas Luebehusen, and Col. W.H. Van Atta for their contributions. The ADRDA, through the personal cooperation of Jerome H. Stone, president, and other professional staff, has given unstinting advice and support in the development of this book.

Hazel E. Carroll, R.N., director of nursing at the Keswick Home, Baltimore, Md., Ruth Lovett, R.N., former assistant director of nursing at Greater Baltimore Medical Center, and Osa Jackson, Ph.D., R.P.T., assistant professor in the Physical Therapy Department of the University of Maryland School of Medicine, have generously shared with us their knowledge and skill in patient care. Robert Katzman, M.D., chairman of the Department of Neurology at the Albert Einstein College School of Medicine, and Miriam Aronson, Ph.D., assistant professor in the departments of Psychiatry and Neurology of the Albert Einstein College School of Medicine, have read the manuscript. Their insights and comments have been most helpful.

We are grateful to the many people who have advised us in areas outside our expertise. Phyllis J. Erlich, Esq., drafted and reviewed the section on legal matters and contributed to the section on financial concerns. Frederick T. DeKuyper, assistant general counsel of The Johns Hopkins University, also read and commented on the chapter on financial and legal matters.

Matthew Tayback, Sc.D., director of the Maryland State Office on Aging, and Susan Coller, director of training and educational development of the Maryland State Office on Aging, provided information about federal and state offices on aging. Nancy P. Whitlock, of the Medical Assistance Policy Administration of the Maryland Department of Health and Mental Hygiene, and Sheridan Gladhill, Richard Strauss, William Coons, and Robert Augustine, of the Health Care Financing Administration, guided us through the complexities

## Acknowledgments

of Medicare and Medicaid policy. Gene VandeKieft, C.I.C., of Rice and Associates, Inc., advised us about insurance. Domenic J. LaPonzina, public affairs officer of the Baltimore District of the Internal Revenue Service, assisted us with tax law. Oliver P. Boyer, Jr., of the Jarrettsville Federal Savings and Loan Association, suggested many of the places to look for financial assets.

Maggie Rider, our secretary, cheered us on, kept the office running smoothly while we wrote and rewrote the manuscript, and provided suggestions about the book's content. Bonnie Strauss and Violet E. Goodman helped with important administrative assistance, and a team of typists saw us through many revisions. We especially appreciate the advice and guidance of our editor, Anders Richter, and the staff of The Johns Hopkins University Press who coordinated and expedited publication.

Family and friends are a special blessing as a book develops. They live with a manuscript on the dining room table, they think up possible titles on their vacation, they encourage, cheer, and endure. They have read the manuscript and shared their vision and their ideas. Our special thanks go to Karen Rabins, Hank Kalapaca, Randy Lang, Catherine Lang, Mr. and Mrs. F. R. Lawson, Eugene Peterson, and Edna Bradford.

# 1

## DEMENTIA

*For two or three years Mary had known that her memory was slipping. First she had trouble remembering the names of her friends' children, and one year she completely forgot the strawberry preserves she had put up. She compensated by writing things down. After all, she told herself, she was getting older. But then she would find herself groping for a word she had always known, and she worried that she was getting senile.*

*Recently, when she was talking with a group of friends, Mary would realize that she had forgotten more than just an occasional name—she lost the thread of the conversation altogether. She compensated for this too: she always made an appropriate answer, even if she secretly felt confused. No one noticed, unless perhaps her daughter-in-law, who said to her best friend, "I think Mother is slipping." It worried Mary—sometimes depressed her—but she always denied that anything was wrong. There was no*

1

one to whom she could say, "I am losing my mind. It is literally slipping away as I watch." Besides, she didn't want to think about it, didn't want to think about getting old, and, most important, she didn't want to be treated as if she were senile. She was still enjoying life and able to manage.

Then in the winter Mary got sick. At first she thought it was only a cold. She saw a doctor, who gave her some pills, and asked her what she expected at her age, which annoyed her. She rapidly got much worse. She went to bed, afraid, weak, and very, very tired. Mary's daughter-in-law got a telephone call from Mary's neighbor. Together they found the old woman semiconscious, feverish, and mumbling incoherently.

During the first few days in the hospital Mary had only an intermittent, foggy notion of what was happening. The doctors told her family that she had pneumonia, and that her kidneys were working poorly. All the resources of a modern hospital were mobilized to fight the infection.

Mary was in a strange place, and nothing was familiar. People, all strangers, came and went. They told her where she was, but she forgot. In strange surroundings she could no longer compensate for her forgetfulness, and the delirium caused by the acute illness aggravated her confusion. She thought her husband came to see her: a handsome young man in his war uniform. Then when her son came, she was surprised that they would come together. Her son kept saying, "But Mom, Dad has been dead for twenty years." But she knew he wasn't, because he had just been there. Then when she complained to her daughter-in-law that she never came, she thought the girl lied when she said, "But Mother, I was just here this morning." In truth, she could not remember the morning.

People came and poked and pushed, and shoved things in and out and over her. They gave her needles and they

2

*wanted her to blow into their bottles. She did not under-
stand and they could not explain that blowing in the bottles
forced her to breathe deeply to strengthen her lungs and
improve her circulation. The bottles became part of her
nightmare. She could not remember where she was. When
she had to go to the bathroom, they put rails on her bed
and refused to let her go, so that she cried and wet herself.*

*Gradually, Mary got better. The infection cleared and the
dizziness passed. Only during the acute phase of her illness
did she imagine things, but after the fever and infection
had passed, the confusion and forgetfulness seemed more
severe than before. Although the illness had probably not
affected the gradual course of her memory loss, it had
weakened her considerably and taken her out of the familiar setting in which she had been able to function. Most
significantly, the illness had focused attention on the seri-
ousness of her situation. Now her family realized she could
no longer live alone.*

*The people around Mary talked and talked. No doubt
they explained their plans, but she forgot. When she was
finally released from the hospital, they took her to her
daughter-in-law's house. They were happy about something
that day, and led her into a room. Here at last were some
of her things, but not all. She thought perhaps the rest of
her things had been stolen while she was sick. They kept
saying they had told her where her things were, but she
couldn't remember what they said.*

*This is where they said she lived now, in her daughter-in-
law's house—except that long ago she had made up her
mind that she would never live with her children. She
wanted to live at home. At home she could find things. At
home she could manage—she believed—as she always had.
At home, perhaps, she could discover what had become of
a lifetime of possessions. This was not her home: her
independence was gone, her things were gone, and Mary*

*felt an enormous sense of loss. Mary could not remember
her son's loving explanation—that she couldn't manage
alone and that bringing her to live in his home was the best
arrangement he could work out for her.*

Often, Mary was afraid, a nameless, shapeless fear. Her
impaired mind could not put a name or an explanation to
her fear. People came, memories came, and then they
slipped away. She could not tell what was reality and what
was memory of people past. The bathroom was not where it
was yesterday. Dressing became an insurmountable ordeal.
Her hands forgot how to button buttons. Sashes hung
inexplicably about her, and she could not think how to
manage them or why they hung there.

Mary gradually lost the ability to make sense out of what
her eyes and ears told her. Noises and confusion made her
feel panicky. She couldn't understand, they couldn't explain,
and often panic overwhelmed her. She worried about her
things: a chair, and the china that had belonged to her
mother. They said they had told her over and over, but she
could not remember where her things had gone. Perhaps
someone had stolen them. She had lost so much. What
things she still had, she hid, but then she forgot where she
hid them.

"I cannot get her to take a bath," her daughter-in-law
said in despair. "She smells." "How can I send her to the
senior center if she won't take a bath?" For Mary the bath
became an experience of terror. The tub was a mystery.
From day to day she could not remember how to manage
the water: sometimes it all ran away, sometimes it kept
rising and rising, so that she could not stop it. The bath
involved remembering so many things. It meant remembering
how to undress, how to find the bathroom, how to wash.
Mary's fingers had forgotten how to unzip zippers; her feet
had forgotten how to step into the tub. There were so many

*things for an injured mind to think about that panic
overwhelmed her.*

How do any of us react to trouble? We might try to get
away from the situation for a while, and think it out. One
person may go out for a beer; another may weed the
garden or go for a walk. Sometimes we react with anger.
We fight back against those who cause, or at least participate in, our situation. Or we become discouraged for a
while, until nature heals us or the trouble goes away.

Mary's old ways of coping with trouble remained. Often
when she felt nervous, she thought of going for a walk. She
would pause on the porch, look out, drift out, and walk
away—away from the trouble. Yet the trouble remained and
now it was worse, for Mary would be lost, nothing would
be familiar: the house had disappeared, the street was not
the one she knew—or was it one from her childhood, or
where they lived when the boys were growing up? The
terror would wash over her, clutching at her heart. Mary
would walk faster.

Sometimes Mary would react with anger. It was an anger
she herself did not understand. But her things were gone,
her life seemed gone. The closets of her mind sprang open
and fell shut, or vanished altogether. Who would not be
angry? Someone had taken her things, the treasures of a
lifetime. Was it her daughter-in-law, or her own mother-in-
law, or a sister resented in childhood? She accused her
daughter-in-law but quickly forgot the suspicion. Her
daughter-in-law, coping with an overwhelming situation,
was unable to forget.

Many of us remember the day we began high school. We
lay awake the night before, afraid of getting lost and not
finding the classrooms the next day in a strange building.
Every day was like that for Mary. Her family began
sending her to an adult day care center. Every day a

busdriver came to pick her up, and every day her daughter-in-law came to get her, but from day to day Mary could not remember that she would be taken home. The rooms were not dependable. Sometimes Mary could not find them. Sometimes she went in the men's bathroom. Sometimes she did not know whether they would come to get her in the evening.

Many of Mary's social skills remained, so she was able to chat and laugh with the other people in the day care center. As Mary relaxed in the center she enjoyed the time she spent there with other people, although she could never remember what she did there well enough to tell her daughter-in-law.

Mary loved music; music seemed to be imbedded in a part of her mind that she retained long after much else was lost. She loved to sing old, familiar songs. She loved to sing at the day care center. Even though her daughter-in-law could not sing well, Mary did not remember that, and the two women discovered that they enjoyed singing together.

The time finally came when the physical and emotional burden of caring for Mary became too much for her family and she went to live in a nursing home. After the initial days of confusion and panic passed, Mary felt secure in her small, sunny bedroom. She could not remember the schedule for the day but the reliability of the routine comforted her. Some days it seemed as if she were still at the day care center, sometimes she was not sure. She was glad the toilet was close by where she could see it and did not have to remember where it was.

Mary was glad when her family came to visit. Sometimes she remembered their names, more often she did not. She never remembered that they had come last week and so she regularly scolded them for abandoning her. They could never think of much to say but they put their arms around her frail body, held her hand, and sat silently or sang old *songs. She was glad when they didn't try to remind her of what she had just said or that they had come last week, or ask her if she remembered this person or that one. She liked it best when they just held her and loved her.*

Someone in your family has been diagnosed as having a dementia. This could be Alzheimer's disease, multi-infarct dementia, or one of several other diseases. Perhaps you are not sure yet which condition it is. Whatever the name of the disease, a person close to you has lost some of his intellectual ability—the ability to think and remember. He may become increasingly forgetful. His personality may appear to change, or he may become depressed, moody, or withdrawn.

Many, although not all, of the disorders that cause these symptoms in adults are chronic and irreversible. When a diagnosis of an irreversible dementia is made, the patient and his family face the task of learning to live with this illness. Whether you decide to care for the person at home or to have him cared for in a nursing home, you will find yourself facing new problems and coping with your feelings about having someone close to you develop an incapacitating illness.

This book is designed to help you with that adjustment and with the tasks of day-to-day management of a chronically ill family member. We have found that there are questions many families ask. This material can help you begin to find answers, but it is not a substitute for the help of your doctor and other professionals.

## WHAT IS DEMENTIA?

You may have discovered that many names have been given to the symptoms of memory loss and loss of thinking and reasoning capacity in adults. This is the result of different descriptions and definitions in older medical books. Commonly used terms include "organic brain syndrome," "senility," "hardening of the arteries," or "chronic brain syndrome."

Your doctor may say "Alzheimer's disease," "multi-infarct disease," "senile dementia," or "presenile dementia." In this book we will refer to these conditions as *dementia*.

Doctors use the word *dementia* in a specific way. It means a loss or impairment of mental powers. It comes from two Latin words, which mean *away* and *mind*. Dementia does not mean crazy. It has been chosen by the medical profession as the least offensive and most accurate term to describe this group of illnesses. *Dementia* describes a group of symptoms and is not the name of a disease or diseases that cause the symptoms.

There are two major conditions that result in the symptoms of mental confusion, memory loss, disorientation, intellectual impairment, or similar problems. These two conditions may look similar to the casual observer and can be confused. (They will be discussed in more detail in Chapter 17.) The first condition, delirium, comprises a group of symptoms in which the person is less alert than normal. He is often drowsy but may fluctuate between drowsiness and restlessness. Like the demented person, he is also confused, disoriented, or forgetful. These conditions have also been called "acute brain syndromes" or "reversible brain syndromes." Delirium can be caused by illnesses such as pneumonia or kidney infection, malnutrition, or reactions to medications.

With the second condition, dementia, there is impaired intellectual functioning in a person who is clearly awake. The symptoms of dementia can be caused by several different diseases. Some of these diseases are treatable, others are not. Thyroid disease, for example, may cause a dementia that can be reversed with correction of a thyroid abnormality. In Chapter 17, we have summarized some of the diseases that can cause dementia.

*Alzheimer's disease* appears to be the most frequent cause of irreversible dementia in adults. The intellectual impairment progresses gradually from forgetfulness to total disability.

Structural changes in the brain are visible in autopsies of people who suffered from Alzheimer's disease. The cause of the illness is not known, and at present physicians know of no way to stop or cure it. However, much can be done to make the patient comfortable and give the family a sense of control of the situation.

*Multi-infarct dementia* is believed to be the second most common cause of irreversible dementia. This is a series of strokes within the brain. Sometimes strokes may be so tiny that neither you nor the afflicted person is aware of any change, but all together they can destroy enough bits of brain tissue to affect memory and other intellectual functions. This condition used to be called "hardening of the arteries," but autopsy studies have shown that it is stroke damage rather than inadequate circulation that causes the problem. In some cases, treatment can reduce the possibility of further damage.

Alzheimer's disease and multi-infarct dementia sometimes occur together. The diagnosis and characteristics of these diseases are discussed in detail in Chapter 17.

People who have dementing illness may also have other illnesses, and their dementia may make them more vulnerable to other health problems. Other illnesses or reactions to medications often cause delirium in people with dementing illnesses. The delirium can make the person's mental functions and behavior worse. It is vital to his general health and to make his care easier to detect and treat other illnesses promptly. It is important to have a doctor who is able to spend time with you and the patient to do this.

Depression is common in older people, and can be the cause of memory loss, confusion, or other changes in mental function. Dementia caused by depression is reversible. The depressed person's memory frequently gets better when the depression is treated. Although depression can also occur in a person with an irreversible dementia, depression should always be treated.

9

Several other uncommon conditions cause dementia. These will be discussed in Chapter 17.

The dementing diseases know no social or racial lines: the rich and the poor, the wise and the simple alike become victims. There is no reason to be ashamed or embarrassed because a family member has a dementing illness. Many brilliant and famous people have suffered from dementing illnesses. Although dementias associated with the final stage of syphilis were common in the past, this is very rare today. There is no other known link between dementia and venereal disease.

Severe memory loss is *never* a normal part of growing older. According to the best studies available, 5 percent of older people suffer from a severe intellectual impairment and a similar number may suffer from milder impairments. The diseases become more prevalent in people who survive into their 80s and 90s, but about 80 percent of those who live into very old age never experience a significant memory loss or other symptoms of dementia. A slight forgetfulness is common as we age but usually is not enough to interfere with our lives. Most of us know elderly people who are active and in full command of their intellect in their 70s, 80s, or 90s. Margaret Mead, Pablo Picasso, Arturo Toscanini, and Duke Ellington all were still active in their careers when they died: all were past 75; Picasso was 91.

As more people in our population live into later life, it becomes crucial that we learn more about dementia. It has been estimated that 2–4 million people in the United States have some degree of intellectual impairment. More than half of the $21.6 billion projected to be spent on nursing home care in 1980 was tied to the care of people with chronic brain disorders.

## THE PERSON WITH A DEMENTING ILLNESS

The person suffering from a dementing illness has difficulty remembering things, although he may be skillful at concealing this. His ability to understand, reason, and use good judgment may be impaired. The onset and the course of the condition depend upon which disease caused the condition and upon other factors, some of which are unknown to researchers. Sometimes the onset of the trouble is sudden: looking back, you may say, "After a certain time, Dad was never himself." Sometimes the onset is gradual: family members may not notice at first that something is wrong. Sometimes the afflicted person himself may be the first to notice something wrong. The person with a mild dementia is often able to describe his problem clearly: "Things just go out of my mind." "I start to explain and then I just can't find the words."

People respond to their problems in different ways. Some people become skillful at concealing the difficulty. Some keep lists to jog their memory. Some vehemently deny that anything is wrong or blame their problems on others. Some people become depressed or irritable when they realize that their memory is failing. Others remain outwardly cheerful. Usually, the person with a mild to moderate dementia is able to continue to do most of the things he has always done. Like a person with any other disease, he is able to participate in his treatment, in family decisions, and in planning for the future.

Early memory problems are sometimes mistaken for stress, depression, or even mental illness. This misdiagnosis creates an added burden for the person and the family.

*A wife recalls the onset of her husband's dementing illness, not in terms of his forgetfulness but in terms of his mood and attitude:*

*"I didn't know anything was wrong. I didn't want to see it.*

11

*Charles was quieter than usual; he seemed depressed, but he blamed it on people at work. Then his boss told him he was being transferred—a demotion, really—to a smaller branch office. They didn't tell me anything. They suggested we take a vacation. So we did. We went to Scotland. But Charles didn't get any better. He was depressed and irritable. After he took the new job, he couldn't handle that either; he blamed it on the younger men. He was so irritable, I wondered what was wrong between us after so many years. We went to a marriage counselor and that only made things worse. I knew he was forgetful but I thought that it was caused by stress.''*

*Her husband said at the time, "I knew something was wrong. I could feel myself getting uptight over little things. People thought I knew things about the plant that I—I couldn't remember. The counselor said it was stress. I thought it was something else, something terrible. I was scared.''*

Some people experience changes in personality. Many of the qualities that a person has always had may remain: he may always have been sweet and lovable and may remain so, or he may always have been a difficult person to live with and may become more so. Other people may change dramatically, from amiable to demanding or from energetic to apathetic. They may become passive, dependent, and listless, or they may become restless, easily upset, and irritable. Sometimes they become demanding, fearful, or depressed.

*A daughter says, "Mother was always the cheerful, outgoing person in the family. I guess we knew she was getting forgetful but the worst thing is that she doesn't want to do anything anymore. She doesn't do her hair, she doesn't keep the house neat, she absolutely won't go out.''*

Often little things enormously upset people with memory problems. Tasks that were previously simple may now be too difficult for a person and he may react to this by becoming upset, angry, or depressed.

*From another family: "The worst thing about Dad is his temper. He used to be easy-going. Now he is always hollering over the least little thing. Last night he told our ten year old that Alaska is not a state. He was hollering and yelling and stalked out of the room. Then when I asked him to take a bath we had a real fight. He insisted he had already taken a bath."*

It is important for those around him to remember that many of the person's behaviors are beyond his control: for example, he may not be able to keep his anger in check or to stop pacing the floor. The changes that occur are not the result of an unpleasant personality grown old: they are the result of damage to the brain and are usually beyond the control of the patient.

In those illnesses in which the dementia is progressive, the person's memory will gradually become worse, and his troubles cannot be concealed. He may become unable to recall what day it is or where he is. He may be unable to do simple tasks such as dressing, and may not be able to put words together coherently. As the dementia progresses, it becomes clear that the damage to the brain affects many functions, including memory, motor functions (coordination, writing, walking), and speaking. The person may have difficulty finding the right name for familiar things and he may become clumsy or walk with a shuffle. The sick person's abilities may fluctuate from day to day or even from hour to hour. This makes it harder for families to know what to expect.

Some people with dementing illnesses have hallucinations (hearing, seeing, or smelling things that are not real). This experience is real to the person experiencing it and can be frightening to family members. Some people become suspicious of others; they may hide things or accuse people of stealing from them. Often they simply mislay things and forget where they put them, and in their confusion think someone has stolen them.

*A son recalls: "Mom is so paranoid. She hides her purse. She hides her money, she hides her jewelry. Then she accuses my wife of stealing it. Now she is accusing us of stealing the silverware. The hard part is that she doesn't seem sick. It's hard to believe she isn't doing this deliberately."*

In the final stages of a progressive dementing illness, so much of the brain has been affected that the person is often confined to bed, unable to control urination and unable to express himself. In the last stages of the illness the patient may require skilled nursing care.

It is important to remember that not all these symptoms will occur in the same person. Your family member may never experience some of these symptoms or may experience others we have not mentioned. The course of the disease and the prognosis vary with the specific disorder and with the individual person.

## WHERE DO YOU GO FROM HERE?

You know or suspect that someone close to you has a dementing illness. Where do you go from here? You will need to take stock of your current situation and then identify what needs to be done to help the impaired person and to make the burdens on yourself bearable. There are many questions you must ask. This book will get you started with the answers.

The first thing you need to know is the cause of the disease and its prognosis. Each disease that causes dementia is different. You may have been given different diagnoses and different explanations of the disease, or you may not know what is wrong with the person. However, you must have a diagnosis and some information about the course of the disease before you or the doctor can respond appropriately to day-to-day problems or plan for the future. It is usually better to know what to expect. Your understanding of the illness can help to dispel fears and worries, and it will help you to plan how best you can help the person with a dementing disease.

You need a physician who is willing and able to devote the time and interest required to care for the patient. Chapter 2 describes how a diagnostic evaluation is done and how to find a physician who will care for the ill person.

Even when the disease itself cannot be stopped, *much can be done to improve the quality of life for the afflicted person and for the family.* Chapters 3 through 9 list many of the problems that families face in caring for a person with a dementing illness and offer suggestions for managing them.

Dementing illnesses vary with the specific diseases and with the individual who is afflicted. You may never face many of the problems discussed in this chapter. You may find it most helpful to skip through these chapters to those sections that apply to you.

The key to coping is common sense and ingenuity. Sometimes a family is too close to the problem to see clearly a way of managing. At other times there is no one more ingenious at solving a difficult problem than the family members themselves. Many of the ideas offered here were developed by family members who have called or written to share them with others. These ideas will get you started.

At some point you may find that you will need additional help in caring for an impaired person. Chapter 10 discusses the kinds of help that may be available and how to locate them.

You and the impaired person are part of a family that needs to work together to cope with this illness. Chapter 11 discusses families and the problems that can arise in families. Chapter 12 discusses your feelings and the effects this illness may have on you. Caring for yourself is important for both you and the confused person who is dependent on you, and is discussed in Chapter 13.

Chapter 14 is written for young people who know someone with a dementing illness. Perhaps, as a parent, you will want to read this section also and plan a time to discuss it with your son or daughter. The entire book is written in such a way that a young person will be able to understand any other sections he may want to read.

Chapter 15 discusses legal and financial matters. Although it may be painful to plan ahead, it is most important to do so. Perhaps now is the time to get started with things you may have been avoiding.

A time may come when the impaired person cannot live alone. Chapter 16 discusses nursing homes and other living arrangements.

Chapter 17 discusses the diseases that cause dementia and explains how they differ from other brain disorders. However, it is written to give you a general understanding of terms and conditions, not as a tool for diagnosis.

Chapter 18 briefly reviews the research into Alzheimer's disease and multi-infarct dementia. The reading list in Appendix 1 refers you to other, more detailed information on research.

You may want to use this handbook to inform others about the diseases that cause dementia. The dementing illnesses affect large numbers of people, but their effects on families and their potential management are sometimes poorly understood by professionals and by the general community. Education does not always have to come from the professional person. You, the family, can effectively inform others. Share what you know about dementia with your physician, nursing home staff, and others. The grassroots education of people by people will help to bring dementia out of the closet and into the light of research. This will result in improved care, improved emotional and financial support, and research to seek cures or preventive measures. Use what you know and use this handbook. You will increase the understanding of those around you, and you will reach families who have been struggling in isolation.

Caring for a person with a dementing illness is not easy. We hope the information in this book will help you, but we know that simple solutions are not yet at hand.

Often the text of this book discusses problems. However, it is important to remember that confused people and their families do still experience joy and happiness. Since dementing illnesses develop slowly, they often leave intact the impaired person's ability to enjoy life and to enjoy other people. When things go badly, remind yourself that no matter how bad the person's memory is, or how strange his behavior, he is still a unique and special human being. We can continue to love a person even after he has changed drastically, and even when we are deeply troubled by his present state.

# 2

## GETTING MEDICAL HELP
## FOR THE IMPAIRED PERSON

THIS BOOK is written for you, the family. It is based on the assumption that you and the sick person are receiving professional medical care. The family and the medical professionals are partners in the care of the impaired person. Neither should be providing care alone. This book is not meant to be a substitute for professional skills. However, we recognize that, at the time of this writing, families may have difficulty finding the kind of medical care they need. Misconceptions about dementia do exist among professionals. Not all physicians or other professionals have the time, interest, or skills to diagnose or care for a person with a dementing illness. As the public becomes better informed about the dementing illnesses this will become a thing of the past.

What should you expect from your physician and other professionals? The first thing is an accurate diagnosis. Once a diagnosis has been made, you will need the ongoing help of a physician and perhaps other professionals to manage the dementing illness, to treat concurrent illnesses, and to help you find the resources you need. This chapter is written as a guide to help you find the best possible medical care in your community.

In the course of a dementing illness you may need the special skills of a physician, a social worker, or a nurse. Each is a highly trained professional whose skills complement those of the others. They can work together first to evaluate the impaired person and then to help you with ongoing care. They may use the skills of other professionals as well.

## THE EVALUATION OF THE PERSON WITH A SUSPECTED DEMENTIA

It is important that a thorough evaluation be made when a person suffers from difficulty in thinking, remembering, or learning or shows changes in personality. A complete evaluation tells you and the doctors several things:

1. the exact nature of the person's illness,
2. whether or not the condition can be reversed or treated,
3. the nature and extent of the disability,
4. the areas in which the person can still function successfully,
5. whether the person has other health problems that need treatment and that might be making her mental problems worse,
6. the social and psychological needs and resources of the sick person and the family or care giver, and
7. the changes you can expect in the future.

Procedures vary depending on the physician or hospital. However, a good evaluation includes a medical and neurological examination, an evaluation of the person's social support system, and an evaluation of her remaining abilities.

The evaluation may begin with a careful examination by a physician. He will take a *detailed history* from someone who knows the person well and from the sick person if possible. This tells the doctor how the person has changed, tells him what symptoms the person has had, and gives him information about other medical conditions. The doctor will also give the person a *physical examination*, which may reveal other health problems. A *neurological examination* (asking the person to balance with her eyes closed, tapping her ankles or knees with a rubber hammer, and other tests) may reveal changes in the functioning of the nerve cells of the brain or spine.

The doctor will also do a *mental status examination*, in which he asks the person questions about the time, date, and place where she is. Other questions test her ability to remember, to concentrate, to do abstract reasoning, to do simple calculations, and to copy simple designs. Each of these reveals problems of function in different parts of the brain. When he does this test, he will take into consideration the person's education and the fact that the person may be nervous.

The doctor will order *laboratory tests,* including a number of blood tests. The *CBC* (complete blood count) detects anemia and evidence of infection, either of which malfunction can cause or complicate a dementing illness. *Blood chemistry tests* check for liver and kidney problems, diabetes, and a number of other conditions. Vitamin B-12 level tests and folate level tests check for vitamin deficiencies, which might cause dementia. *Thyroid studies* evaluate the function of the thyroid gland. Thyroid problems are among the more common reversible causes of dementia. The *VDRL test* can indicate a syphilis infection (syphilis was a common cause of dementia before the discovery of penicillin), but a positive VDRL test does not necessarily indicate that the person has ever had syphilis. The blood tests usually involve inserting one needle, which is no more unpleasant than a pin prick.

The *lumbar puncture* (LP), or spinal tap, is done to rule out infection in the central nervous system (for example, tuberculosis) and it may reveal other abnormalities. It is usually done after a local anesthestic has been injected into the back and has few complications. It may not be done if there is no reason to suspect these conditions.

The *EEG* (electroencephalograph) records the electrical activity present in the brain. It is done by attaching little wires to the head with a pastelike material. It is painless but may confuse the forgetful person. It aids in the diagnosis of delirium and can offer evidence of abnormal brain functioning, but occasionally is normal in a demented person.

The *CAT scan* (computerized axial tomogram) is a sophisticated x-ray that produces a picture of the brain. (Ordinary skull x-rays show primarily the bones, and do not show the brain itself.) Changes compatible with Alzheimer's disease may be visible on a CAT scan, but this diagnosis should not be made on the basis of a CAT scan alone. The CAT scan can find evidence of stroke, multi-infarct dementia, tumors, changes in the flow of the fluid that surrounds the brain, and collections of blood which can put pressure on the brain.

The CAT scan involves lying on a table and placing one's head in an object that looks like a very large hair dryer. It is painless but may confuse an already impaired person. If so, a mild sedative can be prescribed to help the person relax. It is not done on all patients, but is ordered when the doctor needs it. The CAT scan has replaced the *pneumoencephalogram* (PEG), in which air is injected by means of a needle into the sac surrounding the spine. The PEG was an uncomfortable test and sometimes made patients temporarily worse.

For some procedures, such as the lumbar puncture and dye injections for the CAT scan, you will be asked to sign an informed consent form. This lists all the possible side effects of the procedure. Reading this can make the procedure seem alarming and dangerous, but in fact, these are safe procedures.

If you have any concerns about possible side effects, a doctor will explain them to you.

The history, physical and neurological exams, and laboratory tests will identify or rule out each of the known causes of dementia. Other evaluations in addition to the medical assessment are done to understand the person's abilities and help you to plan for the future.

A *psychiatric and psychosocial evaluation* is based on interviews with the person and her family. This provides the basis for the development of a specific plan for the care of the individual. It may be done by the doctor, nurse, or social worker who works with the physician. It includes helping the family evaluate their own emotional, physical, and financial resources, the home in which the person lives, the community resources, and the patient's ability to accept or participate in plans.

An *occupational therapy evaluation* helps to determine how much the person is able to do for herself and what can be done to help her compensate for her limitations. It is done by an occupational, rehabilitation, or physical therapist. These therapists are important members of the health care team. Their skills are sometimes overlooked because in the past they were consulted only in cases where there was the potential for physical rehabilitation. However, they are able to identify the things that the person can still do, and to devise ways to help the person remain as independent as possible. Part of this assessment is an *ADL* (activities of daily living) evaluation. The person is observed in a controlled situation to see if she can manage money, fix a simple meal, dress herself, and perform other routine tasks. If she can do part of these tasks, this is noted. These therapists are familiar with a variety of appliances that can help some people.

*Neuropsychological testing* (also called cortical function testing or psychometric testing) may be done to determine in which areas of mental function the person is impaired and in which she is still independent. This testing takes several hours. The tests evaluate such things as memory, reasoning, coordination, writing, and the ability to express oneself and understand instructions. The testing psychologist will be experienced in making people feel relaxed and will take into consideration differences in education and interests.

The final part of the evaluation is your *discussion with the doctor* and perhaps with other members of the evaluating team. At this time the doctor will explain his findings to you and to the patient if she is able to understand at least part of what is happening.

At this time the doctor should give you a specific diagnosis (he may explain that he cannot be certain) and a general idea of the person's prognosis (again, he may not be able to tell you exactly what to expect). The findings of other tests, such as the ADL, the psychological tests, and the social history, will also be explained to you. You should be able to ask questions and come away with an understanding of the findings of the evaluation. The doctor may make recommendations such as the use of medications or community support services or he may refer you to someone who can advise you about community services. You, he, and the afflicted person may identify specific problems and set up a plan to cope with them.

A complete evaluation may take more than one day. You may want to arrange to spread the evaluation over more than one day so that the patient will not get too tired. It usually takes several days for the laboratories to report their findings to the doctor and for him to put all these data together into a report.

Evaluations may be done either with the patient admitted to the hospital or on an outpatient basis. Several factors, including your insurance coverage, the general health of the patient, and your convenience, affect the decision to do an inpatient or outpatient evaluation.

Sometimes family members and occasionally professionals advise against "putting a confused person through the 'ordeal' of an evaluation." We feel that every person with problems in memory and thinking should be fully evaluated. An evaluation is not an unpleasant ordeal. Staff accustomed to working with demented people are usually gentle and kind. It is important that they make the person as comfortable as possible so that they will be able to measure her best performance.

As we have said, there are many reasons why a person might develop the symptoms of dementia. Some of these are treatable. If a treatable problem is not found because an evaluation is not done, the afflicted person and her family may suffer unnecessarily for years. Certain diseases can be treated if they are found promptly, but can cause irreversible damage if they are neglected.

Even if it is found that a person has an irreversible dementia, the evaluation will give you information about how best to care for the impaired person and how best to manage her symptoms. It gives you a basis upon which to plan for the future and, finally, it is important that you know that you have done all that you can for her.

## FINDING SOMEONE TO DO AN EVALUATION

In some areas it can be difficult to find someone who is interested in doing a thorough evaluation of a person with a suspected dementia. This is changing. Your family physician may do the evaluation or may be able to refer you to a specialist who can do an evaluation, or your local hospital may give you the names of physicians who are interested in evaluating people with dementing illnesses. The teaching hospitals or medical schools in your area may know of people with a special interest in this field. The Alzheimer's Disease and Related Disorders Association (see Appendix 2) may be able to give you the names of physicians in your area.

You can ask the evaluating physician what procedures he uses and why before you schedule an evaluation. If you feel from this preliminary conversation that he is not really interested in dementia, you may want to seek someone else.

How do you decide whether an accurate diagnosis has been made for someone in your family? In the final analysis, you must settle on a doctor whom you trust and who you feel has done all he can, and then rely on his judgment. This is much easier when you understand something about the terminology, the diagnostic procedures, and what is known about the dementias. If you have been given differing diagnoses, discuss this frankly with the doctor. It is important that you feel certain that an accurate diagnosis has been made.

You may hear about people with similar symptoms who are "miraculously" cured, or you may hear statements like "senility can be cured." Considerable confusion has arisen because some of the causes of dementia are reversible and because dementia and delirium are sometimes confused. There are some unscrupulous individuals who offer bogus "cures" for these tragic illnesses. An accurate diagnosis and a doctor you trust can assure you that all that can be done is being done. You can also keep informed about the progress of legitimate research through the Alzheimer's Disease and Related Disorders Association and from the major research institutes.

## MEDICAL TREATMENT AND MANAGEMENT OF DEMENTIA

Dementing illnesses are diseases that require continuing medical attention. The availability of professional services varies. You, the caretaker, will provide much of the coordination of care. However, there are times when you will also need the help of professionals.

## The Physician

You will need a physican who will prescribe and adjust medications, answer your questions, and treat other, concurrent illnesses. The physician who provides continuing care will not necessarily be the specialist who provided the initial evaluation of the person. He may be your family doctor, part of a geriatric team, or someone with a special interest in geriatric medicine. This doctor does not have to be a specialist, although he should be able to work with a neurologist or psychiatrist if necessary. The doctor you select for continuing care must:

1. be willing and able to spend the necessary time with you and the sick person,
2. be knowledgeable about dementing illnesses and the special susceptibility of demented patients to other diseases, medications, and delirium,
3. be easily accessible,
4. if possible, be able to make referrals to physical therapists, social workers, and other professionals.

Not all doctors meet these criteria. Some doctors have large practices and do not have the time to focus on your problems. It is impossible for any one person to keep up with all the advances in medicine, and so some doctors may not be skilled in the specialized care of a person with dementia. Finally, some doctors are uncomfortable caring for people with chronic, incurable diseases. However, no physician should give you a diagnosis without following through with referrals to professionals who can give you the help and follow-up you need. You may have to talk with more than one doctor before you find the one who is right for you. Discuss your needs and expectations honestly with him, and talk over how you can best work with him.

## The Nurse

In addition to the knowledge and experience of a physician you may need the skills of a registered nurse who can work with the physician. The nurse may be the person whom you can reach most easily and who can coordinate the work that you, the doctor, and others do to provide the best possible care. She may be the person who understands the difficulties of caring for a person at home. She can observe the person for changes in her health status which need to be reported to the doctor and she can give you support and counsel. After talking with you, she can identify and help to solve many of the problems you face. She can teach you how to provide practical care for the person (coping with catastrophic reactions, giving baths, helping with eating problems, managing a wheelchair). She can teach you how and when to give medicine and how to know whether it is working correctly. A nurse may be available to come to your home to assess the patient and offer suggestions for simplifying the person's environment and minimizing the effort you need to expend.

A licensed vocational (practical) nurse may also be helpful to you.

Your physician should be able to refer you to a nurse, or you can locate this help by calling your health department or a home health agency such as the Visiting Nurse Association.

Medicare or health insurance may pay for nursing services if they are ordered by a physician. (See p. 198.)

In some areas an occupational therapist or physical therapist may be available to help.

## The Social Worker

Social workers have a unique combination of skills: they know the resources and services in your community and they are skilled in assessing your situation and needs and matching these with available services. Some families think of social workers as "just for the poor." This is not true. They are professionals whose skills in helping you find resources can be invaluable. They can also provide practical counseling and help you and your family think through plans. They can help families work out disagreements over care.

Your physician may be able to refer you to a social worker, or if the sick person is hospitalized, the hospital social worker may be able to help you. The local office on aging may have a social worker on the staff who will help anyone over sixty.

Most communities have family service agencies staffed by social workers. To locate local social service agencies, look in the telephone book yellow pages under "Social Services Organizations" or under the listings for your state and local governments. You can write the national office of the Family Service Association of America (see Appendix 2). They accredit private agencies, and can provide you with the names of your nearest agencies.

Social workers work in a variety of settings, including public social service agencies, some nursing homes, senior citizens centers, public housing projects, and local offices of the state department of health. Sometimes these agencies have special units that serve the elderly. There are social workers in private practice in some communities. Social workers are professionally trained. In many states they must also be licensed or accredited. You should know the qualifications and training of the person you select.

Fees for social services vary, depending on the agency, the services you need, and whether or not you are using other services of that agency (such as a hospital). Some agencies charge according to your ability to pay.

It is important to select a social worker who understands the dementing illnesses.

# 3

## CHARACTERISTIC PROBLEMS
## OF DEMENTIA

IN CHAPTERS 3 through 9 we will discuss many of the problems that families may encounter in caring for a person with a dementing illness. Although as yet nothing can be done to cure some dementing illnesses, it is important to remember that *much can be done to make life easier for you and the person with a dementing illness*. The suggestions we offer come from our clinical experience and from the experiences that family members have shared with us.

Each individual and each family is different. You may never experience many of these problems. The problems you will face are influenced by the nature of the specific disease, by your personality, by the sick person's personality, and, often, by other factors, such as where you live. We do not want you to read through this section as if it were a list of what lies ahead of you. It is a comprehensive list of problem areas for you to use as a reference when a specific problem arises.

The very nature of brain injuries can make them difficult to live with. The brain is a vast, complex, mysterious organ. It is the source of our thoughts, our emotions, and our personality. Injury to the brain can cause changes in emotions, personality, and the ability to reason. Most dementing illnesses do their damage gradually, so the effects are not seen suddenly, as are the effects of a major stroke or head injury. Consequently, the behavior of a person with a dementing illness often seems puzzling in contrast to behaviors due to other illnesses. It is not always evident that many of the visible symptoms (changes in personality, for example) are the result of a disease. Because the sick person often looks well, people may interpret his behavior as "odd" or "crazy" and may not be as understanding of your problems as they would be if he had another, more familiar disease. Increased community education is helping to change this.

## SOME GENERAL SUGGESTIONS

Be informed. The more you know about the nature of dementing illnesses, the more effective you will be in devising strategies to manage behavior problems.

Share your concerns with the patient. When a person is only mildly to moderately impaired, he can take part in managing his problem. You may be able to share with each other your grief and worries. Together you may be able to devise memory aids that will help him remain independent. Mildly impaired people may benefit from counseling that can help them accept and adjust to their limitations.

Try to solve your most frustrating problems one at a time. Families tell us that the day-to-day problems often seem to be the most insurmountable. Getting mother to take her bath or getting supper prepared, eaten, and cleaned up can become daily ordeals. *If you are at the end of your rope, single out one thing that you can change to make life easier, and work on that*. Sometimes changing small things makes a big difference.

Get enough rest. One of the dilemmas families often face is that the care giver may not get enough rest or may not have the opportunity to get away from his care giving responsibilities. This can make the care giver less patient and less able to tolerate irritating behaviors. If things are getting out of hand, ask yourself if this is happening to you. If so, you may want to focus on finding ways to get more rest or more frequent breaks from your care-giving responsibilities. We recognize that this is difficult to arrange. We will discuss this in Chapter 10.

Use your common sense and imagination; they are your best tools. Adaptation is the key to success. If a thing cannot be done one way, ask yourself if it must be done at all. For example, if a person can eat successfully with his fingers but cannot use a fork and spoon appropriately, don't fight the problem; serve as many finger foods as possible. Accept changes. If the person insists on sleeping with his hat on, this is not harmful; go along with it.

Maintain a sense of humor; it will get you through many crises. The sick person is still a person. He needs and enjoys a good laugh too. Sharing your experiences with other families will help you. Surprisingly, these groups of families often find their shared experiences both sad and funny.

Try to establish an environment that allows as much freedom as possible but also offers the structure that confused people often need. Establish a regular, predictable, simple routine for meals, medication, exercising, bedtime, and other activities. Do things the same way and at the same time each day. If you establish regular routines, the person may gradually learn what to expect. Change routines only when they aren't working. Keep the person's surroundings reliable and simple. Leave furniture in the same place. Put away clutter.

Remember to talk *to* the confused person. Speak calmly

and gently. Make a point of telling him what you are doing and why. Let him have a part in deciding things as much as possible. Avoid talking *about* him in front of him, and remind others to do this also.

Have an ID necklace or bracelet made for the confused person. Include on it the nature of his disease (e.g., "memory impaired") and your telephone number. This is one of the single most important things you can do. Many confused people get lost or wander away at one time or another and an ID can save you hours of frantic worry.

Keep the impaired person active but not upset. Families often ask if retraining, reality orientation, or keeping active will slow down or stop the course of the disease. Likewise, they may ask if being idle hastens the course of the disease. Some people with dementing illnesses become depressed, listless, or apathetic. Families often wonder whether encouraging such a person to do things will help him to function better.

The relationship of activity to the course of dementing illnesses is not clear. Research continues in this area. Activity helps to maintain physical well-being and may help to prevent other illnesses and infections. Being active helps the ill person to continue to feel that he is involved in the family and that his life has meaning.

It is clear that people with dementing illnesses cannot learn as well as before because brain tissue has been damaged or destroyed. It would be unrealistic to expect them to learn new skills. However, some individuals can learn simple tasks or facts if they are repeated often enough. Some impaired people who feel lost in a new place eventually "learn" their way around.

At the same time, too much stimulation, activity, or pressure to learn may upset the confused person, may upset you, and may accomplish nothing. The key to this is balance:

1. Accept that lost skills are gone for good (the woman who has lost the ability to cook will not learn to fix a meal), *but* know that repeatedly and gently giving information within the person's abilities will help him function more comfortably (the person going into a strange day care setting · will benefit from frequent reminders of where he is).

2. Know that even small amounts of excitement—visitors, laughter, changes—can upset the confused person, *but* plan interesting, stimulating things within his capabilities—a walk, visiting one old friend.

3. Look for ways to simplify activities so that a person can continue to be involved within the limits of his abilities (the woman who can no longer fix a whole meal may still be able to peel the potatoes).

4. Look for things the person is still able to do and focus on them. A person's intellectual abilities are not all lost at once. Both of you will benefit from carefully assessing what he can still do and making the best use of those abilities. For example,

*Mrs. Baldwin often cannot remember the words for things she wants to say but she can make her meaning clear with gestures. Her daughter helps her by saying, "point to what you want."*

## MEMORY PROBLEMS

People with dementing illnesses forget things quickly. For the person with a memory impairment, life may be like constantly coming into the middle of a movie: one has no idea what happened just before what is happening now. People with dementing illnesses may say they will call a friend and forget to do so, may start to prepare a meal and forget to turn the stove off, may forget what time it is or where they are. This forgetfulness of recent events can seem puzzling when the person seems to be able to remember clearly events long past. There are some specific suggestions for memory aids throughout this book. You may think of others that will help you.

Forgetful people may remember events long past more clearly than recent events or they may remember some things and not others. This has to do with the way the brain stores and receives information; *it is not something the person does deliberately.* The success of memory aids depends on the severity of the dementia. A mildly demented person may devise reminders for himself, while a severely impaired person will only become more frustrated by his inability to use the aid. People who are able to read can do chores if you write out instructions. Writing down names and often-used phone numbers also helps. If you are going out, write down where you are going. If you will be gone at mealtime, leave a written reminder to eat.

Have clocks and calendars in view to help the confused person remember what time it is. Mark off the days as they pass. It is often helpful to put a simple list of the day's activities where the person can easily see it. A regular daily routine is much less confusing than frequent changes.

Leave familiar objects (pictures, magazines, TV, radio) in their usual places where the person can see them easily. A tidy, uncluttered house will be less confusing to an impaired person and misplaced items will be easier to find. Some families have found that putting labels on things helps. Labeling drawers "Mary's socks," "Mary's nightgowns" may help.

Remember, however, that with progressive dementing illnesses the person will eventually be unable to read or will not be able to make sense out of what he reads. He may be able to read the words but unable to act on them. Some families then use pictures instead of written messages. For example, it may help to put a picture of a toilet on the bathroom door if the person is in an unfamiliar place or has trouble remembering where the bathroom is.

People are often more confused at night and may get lost going to the bathroom. Strips of reflector tape on the wall from the bedroom to the bathroom help. Night lights will help him see where he is.

Pictures of family members and close friends may help the more confused person remind himself of who these people are. If you are visiting someone in a nursing home, you might try taking along a family picture album. Looking at the pictures may stir bits of pleasant memory in the confused mind.

## OVERREACTING OR CATASTROPHIC REACTIONS

*Even though Miss Ramirez had told her sister over and over that today was the day to visit the doctor, her sister would not get in the car until she was dragged in, screaming, by two neighbors. All the way to the doctor's office she shouted for help and when she got there she tried to run away.*

*Mr. Lewis suddenly burst into tears as he tried to tie his shoelaces. He threw the shoes in the wastebasket and locked himself, sobbing, in the bathroom.*

*Mrs. Coleman described several incidents similar to this one, where her husband had mislaid his glasses.*

*"You threw out my glasses," he told her.*

*"I didn't touch your glasses," she answered.*

*"That's what you always say," he responded. "How do you explain that they are gone?"*

*"You do this to me every time you lose your glasses."*

*"I did not lose them. You threw them out."*

*Reflecting back, Mrs. Coleman knew that her husband had changed. In the past he would have merely asked her if she knew where his glasses were instead of accusing her and starting an argument.*

People with brain diseases often become excessively upset and may experience rapidly changing moods. Strange situations, confusion, groups of people, noises, being asked several questions at once, or being asked to do a task that is difficult for them can precipitate these reactions. The person may weep, blush, or become agitated, angry, or stubborn. He may strike out at those trying to help him. He may cover his distress by denying what he is doing or by accusing other people of things.

When a situation overwhelms the limited thinking capacity of a brain-injured person, he may overreact. Normal people sometimes do this when they are bombarded with more things at one time than they can manage. Impaired people have the same reaction to simpler, everyday experiences. For example,

*Every evening Mrs. Hamilton gets upset and refuses to take a bath. When her daughter insists, she argues and shouts. This makes the rest of the family tense. The whole routine is dreaded by everyone.*

Taking a bath actually means that Mrs. Hamilton must think about several things at once; undressing, unbuttoning, finding the bathroom, turning on faucets, and climbing in a tub. At the same time she feels insecure without clothes on and she feels she has lost her privacy and independence. This is overwhelming for a person who cannot remember doing the thing before, who can't remember how to do all these tasks, and whose mind cannot process all these activities at once. One way to react to this is to refuse to take a bath.

We use the term *catastrophic reaction* to describe this behavior. (The word *catastrophic* is used in a special sense; it does not mean that these situations are necessarily very dramatic or violent.) *Often a catastrophic reaction does not look like behavior caused by a brain illness. The behavior may look as if the person is merely being obstinate, critical, or overemotional.* It may seem inappropriate to get so upset over such a little thing.

Catastrophic reactions are upsetting and exhausting for you and for the confused person. They are especially upsetting when it seems as if the person you are trying to help is being stubborn or critical. The person may get so upset that he refuses necessary care. Learning how to avoid or lessen catastrophic reactions is a major key to easier management of them.

Sometimes catastrophic reactions and forgetfulness are the first behaviors family members see when they begin to realize that something is wrong. The mildly impaired person may benefit by being reassured that his panic is not unusual and that you understand his fear.

The things that help to prevent or reduce catastrophic reactions depend on the individual, on you, and on the extent of his limitations. You will gradually learn how to avoid or limit these reactions. *First, you must fully accept that these behaviors are not just stubbornness or nastiness but a response the person with a dementing illness cannot help.* If you are in doubt, give strong consideration to the possibility that the behavior is beyond the control of the impaired person.

Aids that remind the confused person about what is going on, such as following familiar routines, leaving things in familiar places, and written instructions (for people who can manage them), help to reduce catastrophic reactions. Because catastrophic reactions are precipitated by having to think of several things at once, simplify what the confused person has to think about. Take things one step at a time, and give instructions or information one step at a time. For example, when you help a person bathe, tell the person one thing at a time. Say, "I'm going to unbutton your blouse" and then reassure her, "It's all right." Say, "Now I'm going to slip your blouse off. That's fine. You're a big help. Now take a step up into the tub. I will hold your arm."

Give the confused person time to respond. He may react slowly and become upset if you rush him. Wait for him. If a person is having frequent catastrophic reactions, try to reduce the confusion around him. This might mean having fewer people in the room, having less noise, turning off the TV, or reducing the clutter in the room. The key is to simplify, to reduce the number of signals the impaired, disoriented brain must sort out.

Plan things the impaired person can realistically do. If strange places upset him, you may not want to take him on a trip. If he gets tired or upset quickly, plan shorter visits with friends.

You can avert some catastrophic reactions by simplifying the task facing the impaired person. Mr. Quinn's family recognized that tying shoelaces had become too difficult for him but that he needed to remain as independent as possible. Buying him slip-on shoes solved the problem. Mrs. Coleman's husband often lost things because he forgot where he put them. She found it helpful to ignore his accusations and help him find his glasses. Knowing that accusing her was his way of reacting to his forgetfulness made it easier for her to accept the insult.

When the person does become upset or resistant, remain calm and remove him from the situation in a quiet, unhurried way. Often the emotional storm will be over as quickly as it began and the confused person usually will be relieved that the upset is over. His short memory may work to your advantage: he may quickly forget the trouble.

Try not to express your frustration or anger to the confused person. Your frustration will further upset him when he cannot understand your reaction. Speak calmly. Take things one step at a time. Move slowly and quietly. Remember that the person is *not* being obstinate or doing this intentionally. Avoid trying to reason or argue with an upset individual; this only adds to his confusion and increases his overreaction.

Gently holding a person's hand or patting him may help calm him. Some people respond to being slowly rocked. Try putting your arms around him and rocking back and forth. Some people will be soothed by this but others may feel that your arms are restraining them and will become more upset. Physically restraining a person often adds to his panic. Restrain a person only if it is absolutely essential and if nothing else works.

You may lose your temper with a person who is having catastrophic reactions or is unable to do what seems like a simple task. If you do lose your temper, it usually will make the person's behavior worse. Occasionally losing your temper is not a calamity; take a deep breath and try to approach the problem calmly. The person will probably forget your anger much more quickly than you will.

The most important thing, with this and other situations, is not to let yourself get frustrated and discouraged, but to try to examine thoughtfully what is happening. Try to identify exactly what is upsetting the confused person, and consider how you can change that.

## PROBLEMS WITH SPEECH AND COMMUNICATION

You may have problems understanding or communicating verbally with the impaired person. There are two kinds of problems of communication: the problems a person with a dementing illness has in expressing himself to others, and the problems he has in understanding what people say to him.

## Problems the Impaired Person Has in Making Himself Understood

The nature of communication problems and whether or not they will get worse depend on the specific disease. Do not assume that things will get worse.

Some people have only occasional difficulty finding words. They may have trouble remembering the names of familiar objects or people. They may substitute a word that sounds similar, such as saying "tee" for "tie" or "wrong" for "ring." They may substitute a word with a similar meaning, such as saying "wedding" for "ring" or "music thing" for "piano." They may describe the object they cannot name, such as "it's a thing that goes around" for "ring" or "it's to dress up" for "necktie." Such problems usually do not interfere with your ability to understand what the person means.

Some people have difficulty communicating their thoughts.

*Mr. Zuckerman was trying to say that he had never had a neurological examination before. He said, "I really have not, not really, ever have been done, I have never . . ."*

In some language problems the person cannot communicate the whole thought but he can express a few of the words in the thought.

*Mr. Mason wanted to say that he was worried about missing his ride home. He could only say, "Bus, home."*

Sometimes people are able to ramble on quite fluently, and it seems as if they are talking a lot. They will often string together commonly used phrases, so what they say at first seems to make sense, but upon reflection the listener may not be sure he understood the thought being expressed.

*Mrs. Simmons said, "If I tell you something, I might stop in the middle and . . . I'll be real sure about what I've done, . . . said, . . . that. In past records . . . I can be so much more sure of the . . . After I get my bearing again I can just go on as if nothing happened. We thought it was high time to start remembering. I just love to . . . have to . . . talk."*

In these examples, it is possible to understand what the person is saying if we know the context.

When the limitations in ability to communicate frustrate the confused person and frustrate you, they can lead to a series of catastrophic reactions. For example, the impaired person may burst into tears or stamp out of the room when no one understands him.

Sometimes a person is able to conceal language problems. When a doctor asks a person if he knows the word for a wristwatch (a common question used to evaluate language problems), the patient may say, "Of course I do. Why do you ask?" "I don't want to talk about it. Why are you bothering me?" when he cannot think of the word.

In severe language problems, the person may remember only a few key words, such as "No," which he may use whether or not he means it. Eventually the person may be unable to speak. He may repeat a phrase, cry out intermittently, or mumble unintelligible phrases. In some language problems there seems to be no meaning in the jumbled words the person produces. Family members and care givers often grieve when this happens and they can no longer communicate verbally with a loved one. We sense that language is the most human of mental skills. In some families the person continues to be a friend and companion—although a forgetful one—for a long time, but when he is unable to communicate anymore, the family feels they have lost that companionship. You may worry that the person will be sick or in pain and unable to tell you.

How you help the impaired person communicate depends on the kind of difficulty he is having. If he has been diagnosed as having had a stroke that interferes with language function, he should be seen by a stroke rehabilitation team as soon as he has recovered from the acute phase of his illness. Much can be done to rehabilitate stroke victims.

If the person is having difficulty finding the right word, it is usually less frustrating for him to have you supply the word for him than it is to let him search and struggle for the word. When he uses the wrong word and you know what he means, it may be helpful to supply the correct word. However, if doing so upsets him, it may be best to ignore it. When you don't know what he means, ask him to describe it or point to it. For example, the nurse did not know what Mrs. Kealey meant when she said, "I like your wrong." If the nurse had said, "What?" Mrs. Kealey might have become frustrated in trying to express herself. Instead, the nurse asked, "Describe a wrong." Mrs. Kealey said, "It's a thing that goes around." "Point to it," said the nurse. Mrs. Kealey did and the nurse responded, "Oh, yes, my ring."

When a person is having trouble expressing an idea, you may be able to guess what they want to say. *Ask* them if you are guessing correctly. You might guess wrong, and if you act on an erroneous guess you will add to the confused person's frustration. Say, "Are you worried about catching the bus home?" or "Are you saying you have never had an examination like this before?"

When you cannot communicate in other ways, you can often guess what a person is trying to tell you. Remember that his feeling is usually accurate, although it may be exaggerated or not appropriate to the actual situation, but that his explanation of why he feels a certain way may be confused. If Mr. Mason says, "Bus, home," and you say, "You aren't going on the bus," you will not have responded to his feelings. If you correctly guess that he is worried about going home, you can reassure him by saying, "Your daughter is coming for you at 3:00."

If a person can still say a few words, or shake or nod his head, you will need to ask him simplified questions about his needs. Say "Do you hurt?" "Does this hurt?" Point to a body part rather than name it.

When a person cannot communicate, you must establish a regular routine of checking his comfort. Make sure that clothing is comfortable, that the room is warm, that there are no rashes or sores on his skin, that he is taken to the toilet on a regular schedule, and that he is not hungry or sleepy.

## Problems the Impaired Person Has in Understanding Others

Often people with brain impairments have difficulty comprehending or understanding what you and others tell them. This is a problem that families sometimes misinterpret as uncooperative behavior. For example, you may say, "Mother, I am going to the grocery store. I will be back in half an hour. Do you understand?" Your mother may say, "Oh yes, I understand," when in fact she does not understand at all and will get upset as soon as you are out of sight.

People with dementing illnesses also quickly forget what they did understand. When you give them a careful explanation, they may forget the first part of the explanation before you get to the rest of it.

People with dementing illnesses may have trouble understanding written information even when they can still read the letters or words. For example, to determine exactly what a person can still do, we may hand him a newspaper and have him read the headline, which he may be able to do correctly. Then when we hand him the written instructions "close your eyes" he will not close his eyes, although he may correctly read the words aloud.

At home you may put a note on the refrigerator which says, "Your lunch is in the red bowl." You know the person can read the note but he doesn't eat his lunch. This can be infuriating until you consider that reading and understanding are two different skills, one of which may be lost without the loss of the other. It is not safe to assume that a person can understand and act upon messages he can hear or read. You will need to observe him to know whether he *does* act upon them.

The person who can understand what he is told in person may not be able to comprehend what he is told over the telephone. When a person with a dementing illness does not understand what you told him, the problem is not inattentiveness or willfulness, but an inability of the malfunctioning brain to make sense out of the words it hears.

There are several ways to improve your verbal communication with a person who has a dementing illness.

1. Make sure he does hear you. Hearing acuity declines in later life and many older people have a hearing deficit.
2. Lower the tone (pitch) of your voice. A raised pitch is a nonverbal signal that one is upset. A lower pitch also is easier for the hearing impaired to hear.
3. Eliminate distracting noises or activities. Both because of the possible hearing deficit and because of the impaired person's inability to sort things out, he may be unable to understand you when there are other noises or distractions around him.
4. Use short words and short, simple sentences. Avoid complex sentences. Instead of saying, "I think I'll take the car to the garage tonight instead of in the morning because in the morning I will get caught in traffic," just say, "I'm going to take the car to the garage now."
5. Ask only *one* simple question at a time. If you repeat the question, repeat it exactly. Avoid questions like this,

"Do you want an apple or pie for dessert or do you want to have dessert later?" Complex choices may overload the person's decision-making ability.

6. Ask the person to do one task at a time, not several. He may not be able to remember several tasks or may be unable to make sense out of your message. Most of the things we ask a person to do—take a bath, get ready for bed, put on a coat so we can go to the store—involve several tasks. The impaired person may not be able to sort out these tasks. We help him by breaking down each project into individual steps and asking the person to do one step at a time.

7. Speak slowly, and wait for the person to respond. The impaired person's response may be much slower than what seems natural to us. Wait.

You can improve communication with the person and your understanding of his needs without the usual forms of conversation. People communicate through both what they say and the way they move their face, eyes, hands, and bodies. Everyone uses this nonverbal system of communication without thinking about it. For example, we say, "he looks mad," "you can tell by the way they look at each other that they are in love," "you can tell by the way he walks who's boss," "I know you aren't listening to me," etc. These are all things we are communicating without words. Brain-impaired people can remain sensitive to these nonverbal messages when they cannot understand language well, and they often remain able to express themselves nonverbally.

For example, if you are tired, you may send nonverbal messages that upset the impaired person. Then he may get agitated, which will upset you. Your hands, face, and eyes will reveal your distress, which further agitates the confused person. If you are unaware of the significance of body language, you may wonder what happened to get him upset.

In fact, we all do this all the time. For example, "No, I am not upset," you tell a spouse. "But I know you are," he replies. He can tell by the set of your shoulders that you are upset.

If you are living with a person suffering from dementia, you have already learned to identify many of the nonverbal clues that he sends to make his needs known. Here are some additional ways to communicate nonverbally:

1. Remain pleasant, calm, and supportive. (Even if you feel upset, your body language will help to keep the confused person calm.)
2. Smile, take the person's hand, put an arm around his waist, or in some other physical way express affection.
3. Look directly at him. *Look* to see if the person is paying attention to you. If he uses body language to signal that he is not paying attention, try again in a few minutes.
4. Use other signals besides words: point, touch, hand the person things. Demonstrate an action or describe it with your hands (for example, brushing teeth). Sometimes if you get him started he will be able to continue the task.
5. Avoid assuming complex reasons for the person's behavior. Because the person's brain can no longer process information properly, he experiences the world around and within differently from the way you see things. Since nonverbal communication depends on a whole different set of skills from verbal communication, you may be better able to understand him by considering what it *feels* like he is saying rather than what you *think* he is saying, either through actions or words.

Even when a person is severely confused and unable to communicate, he or she still needs and enjoys affection. Holding hands, hugging, or just sitting companionably together is an important way to continue to communicate. The physical care that you give a severely impaired person communicates to him your concern and that he is protected.

## LOSS OF COORDINATION

Because dementing illnesses affect many parts of the brain, the person with a dementia may lose the ability to make his hands and fingers do certain familiar tasks. He may understand what he wants to do, and although his hands and fingers are not stiff or weak, the message just does not get through from the mind to the fingers. Doctors use the word *apraxia* to describe this. An early sign of apraxia is a change in the person's handwriting. Another, later indication is a change in the way a person walks. Apraxias may progress gradually or change abruptly, depending on the disease. For example, at first a person may seem only slightly unsteady when walking but he may gradually change to a slow, shuffling gait.

It can be difficult for the person not trained to evaluate dementing illnesses to separate problems of memory (can the person remember what he is supposed to do?) from problems of apraxia (can the person not make his muscles do what they are supposed to do?). Both problems occur when the brain is damaged by the disease. It is not always necessary to distinguish between them in order to help the person manage as independently as possible.

When apraxia begins to affect walking, the person may be slightly unsteady. You must watch for this and provide either a handrail or someone to hold on to when the person is using stairs and stepping up onto or down off of a curb.

Losses of coordination and manual skills may lead to problems in daily living such as bathing, managing buttons or zippers, dressing, pouring a glass of water, and eating. Dialing a telephone requires good coordination, and a person who does not appear to have any motor impairment may in fact be unable to dial a telephone to call for help. A pushbutton telephone may help, but it may also be difficult for the confused person to learn the new skill of using a touch-tone phone.

Some of the things a person has difficulty with may have to be given up. Others can be modified so that the impaired person can remain partially independent. When you modify a task, the key is to simplify, rather than change, the task. Because of his intellectual impairment, the person with a dementing illness may be unable to learn a new, simpler task. Consider the nature of each task. Ask yourself if it can be done in a simpler way. For example, shoes that slip on are easier than shoes with laces. Soup is easier to drink out of a mug than to spoon from a bowl. Finger foods are more easily managed than things that must be cut with knife and fork. Can the person do part of the task if you do the difficult part? You may already have discovered that the person can dress himself if you help with buttons or snaps.

A person may feel tense, embarrassed, or worried about his clumsiness. He may try to conceal his increasing disability by refusing to participate in activities. For example,

*Mrs. Fisher had always enjoyed knitting. When she abruptly gave up this hobby her daughter could not understand what had happened. Mrs. Fisher said only that she no longer liked to knit. In fact, her increasing apraxia was making knitting impossible, and she was ashamed of her awkwardness.*

A relaxed atmosphere often helps make the person's clumsiness less apparent. It is not unusual for a person to have more difficulty with a task when he is feeling tense.

Sometimes a person can do something one time and not another time. This may be a characteristic of the brain impairment and not laziness. Being hurried, being watched, being upset, or being tired can affect a person's ability to do things—just as it does to a normal person. Having a brain disease makes these natural fluctuations more dramatic. Sometimes people can do one task with no problem, such as zipping up trousers, and be unable to do another similar task, such as zipping up a jacket. It may seem that the person is being difficult, but the reason may actually be that one task is impossible because it is different in some way.

Sometimes a person can do a task if you break it down into a series of smaller tasks and tell him to do each step. For example, brushing your teeth involves picking up the toothbrush, putting the toothpaste on it, putting the toothbrush in your mouth, brushing, rinsing, etc. Gently remind the person of each step. It may help to demonstrate. You may have to repeat each step several times. Sometimes it helps to put a familiar tool, such as a spoon or comb, into the person's hand and gently start his arm moving in the right direction. Beginning the motion seems to help the brain remember the task.

An occupational therapist is trained to assess the motor skills the person has retained and how he may make the best use of them. If you have access to an occupational therapy evaluation, this information can help you give the confused person the help he needs without taking away his independence.

In the later stages of some of the dementing diseases, extensive loss of muscle control occurs and the person may bump into things and fall down. This will be discussed in Chapter 5.

People with dementing illnesses may have other diseases as well that interfere with their ability to do daily tasks. Part of the problem may be in the muscles or joints and another part of the problem in the impaired brain. Such complicating conditions include tremors (shaking), muscle weakness, joint or bone diseases such as arthritis, or stiffness caused by medications.

There are many techniques and devices to help people with physical limitations remain independent. When you consider such techniques or devices, remember that most of them require the ability to learn to do something a new way or to learn to use a new gadget. People with dementing illnesses may not be able to learn the new skills needed.

Some people have tremors. These are shaking movements of the hands or body. These can make many activities difficult for a person, but an occupational therapist or physical therapist may be able to show you how to minimize the effects of tremors.

Some people with neurological conditions, especially Parkinson's disease, have difficulty starting a movement or may get "stuck" in the middle of a movement. This can be frustrating for both of you. If this is a problem, here are some helpful hints:

1. If the person becomes "glued" to the floor while walking, tell him to walk toward a goal or object. This may help him get going again.
2. It may be easier to get out of a chair that has armrests. Raise the sitting person's center of gravity by raising the chair seat two to four inches. A firm seat is needed. Use a firm pillow or a higher chair such as a dining room chair or a director's chair. Avoid low chairs with soft cushions. Instruct the person to move forward to the edge of the chair and spread his feet about one foot apart to give a wider base to stand on. Ask the person to put his hands on the armrests and then to rock back and forth to gain momentum. On the count of 3, have him get up quickly. Have him take time to get his balance before he begins to walk.
3. Sitting down in a chair may be easier to do when the person puts his hands on the arm rests, bends forward as far as possible, and sits down slowly.

Muscle weakness or stiffness may occur when a person does not move around much. Exercise is important for memory-impaired people.

Occasionally a person who is taking one of the major tranquilizers or neuroleptic drugs will get stiff and rigid or may become restless. These may be side effects of the medication. They can be very uncomfortable. Notify your doctor. He can change the dosage or give another medication to overcome this effect.

## LOSS OF SENSE OF TIME

The uncanny ability normal individuals have for judging the passage of time is one of the first losses of a dementia patient. He may repeatedly ask you what time it is, feel that you have left him for hours when you are out of sight for a few minutes, or want to leave a place as soon as he has arrived. It is not hard to understand this behavior when you consider that in order to know how much time has passed, one must be able to remember what one has done with the immediate past. The person who forgets quickly has no way to measure the passage of time.

In addition to this defect of memory, it appears that dementing diseases can affect the internal clock that keeps the rest of us on a reasonably regular schedule of sleeping, waking, and eating. It will be helpful to you to recognize that this behavior is not deliberate (although it can be irritating). It is the result of the loss of brain function.

The ability to read a clock may be lost early in the course of the disease. Even when a person can look at the clock and say, "It is 3:15," he may be unable to make sense out of this information.

Not being able to keep track of time can worry the forgetful person. Many of us, throughout our lives, are dependent upon a regular time schedule. Not knowing the time can make a person worry that he will be late, be forgotten, miss the bus, overstay his welcome, miss lunch, or miss his ride home. The confused person may not know just what he is worried about, but a general feeling of anxiety may make him ask you what time it is. And, of course, as soon as you answer him, he will forget the whole conversation, and ask again.

Sometimes a person feels that you have deserted him when you have been gone only briefly. This is because he cannot remember. Sometimes setting a timer or an old-fashioned hourglass will help these people wait more patiently for your return. Perhaps you can think of other ways to reduce this behavior. For example,

*When Mr. and Mrs. Jenkins went to dinner at their son's house, Mr. Jenkins would almost immediately put his hat and coat on and insist that it was time to go home. When he could be persuaded to stay for the meal, he insisted on leaving immediately afterward. His son thought he was just being rude.*

Things went more smoothly when the family understood that this was because the unfamiliar house, the added confusion, and Mr. Jenkins's lost sense of time upset him. The family thought back over Mr. Jenkins's life and hit upon an old social habit that helped them. In earlier years, he had enjoyed watching the football game after Sunday dinner. Now his son turned on the TV as soon as Mr. Jenkins finished eating. Since this was an old habit, Mr. Jenkins would stay for about an hour, giving his wife time to visit, before he got restless for home.

# 4

## PROBLEMS IN INDEPENDENT LIVING

AS A PERSON BEGINS to develop a dementing illness, she may begin to have difficulty managing independently. You may suspect that she is mismanaging her money, worry that she should not be driving, or wonder if she should be living alone. People with dementing illnesses often appear to be managing well, and they may insist that they are fine and that you are interfering. It can be difficult to know when you should take over and how much you should take over. It can also be painful to take away these outward symbols of a person's independence, or the confused person may adamantly refuse to move, to stop driving, or to relinquish her financial responsibilities.

Part of the reason that making these changes is so difficult is because they symbolize giving up independence and responsibility and therefore all of the family members may have strong feelings about them. (We will discuss these role

55

changes in Chapter 11.) Making necessary changes will be easier when you understand the feelings involved.

The first step in deciding whether the time has come to make changes in a person's independence is to get an evaluation. This will tell you what the person is still able to do and what she is no longer able to do, and it will give you the authority to insist upon necessary changes. When a professional evaluation is not available, you and your family must analyze each task as thoroughly and objectively as possible, and decide whether the person can still do specific tasks *completely, safely,* and *without becoming upset.*

A dementing illness brings about many kinds of losses. It means losing control over one's daily activities, losing independence, losing skills, and losing the ability to do those things that make one feel useful or important. A dementing illness limits the possibilities the future can hold. While others can look forward to things getting better, the ill person must gradually realize that her future is limited. Perhaps the most terrible loss of all is the loss of memory. Losing one's memories means losing one's day-to-day connections with others and with one's past. The far past may seem like the present. Without a memory of today or an understanding that the past is past, the future ceases to have meaning.

As losses accumulate in anyone's life, it is natural for him or her to cling even more tightly to the things that remain. Understandably, a confused person might respond to such changes with resistance, denial, or anger. The confused person's need for familiar surroundings and the determination of most people not to be a burden on anyone make it understandable that the disabled person will not want to give up these things. To accept that, she would have to face the extent and finality of her illness, which she may not be able to do.

In addition, the person may be unable to make complete sense out of what is going on. If she is not able to assess her own limitations, it may seem to her as if things are being unfairly taken away from her and that her family is "taking over." By recognizing how she may feel, you may be able to find ways to help her make the necessary changes and still feel that she is in control of her life.

## WHEN A PERSON MUST GIVE UP A JOB

The time when the person must give up a job depends on the kind of job she has and whether she must drive as part of her job. Sometimes an employer will tell you or the impaired person that she must retire. Some employers will be willing to maintain a person in a job that is not too demanding. Sometimes the family must make this decision. You may realize that this time has come.

If the person must give up her job, there are two areas that you must consider: the emotional and psychological adjustments involved in such a major change, and the financial changes that will be involved. A person's job is a key part of her sense of who she is. It helps her to feel that she is a valued member of society. The impaired person may resist giving up her job or may deny that anything is wrong. Her adjustment to retirement may be a painful and distressing time. If these things happen a counselor or social worker can be invaluable in helping you.

It is important that you consider the financial future of the impaired person. (This will be discussed in Chapter 15.) Retirement can create special problems. Individuals who are forced to retire early because of a dementing illness should be entitled to the same retirement and disability benefits as a person with any other disabling *disease*. In some cases, disability benefits have been denied on the erroneous grounds that "senility" is not a disease and the impaired person has been forced to resign or take an early retirement. This can substantially reduce her income. If this happens, you may want to obtain legal counsel.

The Disability Division of the Social Security Administration requires that a person transfer her skills to a similar, less demanding job. The demented person, although she may have good skills remaining, may be unable to learn a new job. If she is denied benefits for this reason, you may want to seek legal advice.

## WHEN A PERSON CAN NO LONGER MANAGE MONEY

The impaired person may be unable to balance her checkbook, she may be unable to make change, or she may become irresponsible with her money. Occasionally, when a person can no longer manage her money, she may become nasty and accuse others of stealing from her.

*Said Mr. Fried, "My wife has kept the books for the family business for years. I knew something was wrong when my accountant came to me and told me the books were a terrible mess."*

*Mr. Rogers said, "My wife was giving money to the neighbors, hiding it in the waste basket, and losing her purse. So I took her purse—and her money—away from her. Then she was always saying I stole her money."*

Since money often represents independence, sometimes people are unwilling to give up control of their finances.

You may be able to take over the household accounts by simply correcting the person's efforts. If you have to take the person's checkbook away against her wishes it may help to write down a memo such as "my son John now takes care of my checkbook" and put this note where the confused person can refer to it to refresh her memory.

It can be upsetting when a person accuses others of stealing, but this is easier to understand when you think about human nature. We have been taught all our life to be careful with money and when money disappears most of us wonder if it was stolen. As a person's brain becomes less able to remember what is really happening, it is not surprising that she becomes anxious and suspicious that her money is being stolen. Avoid getting into arguments about it, since they may upset her more.

Some families find that giving the forgetful person a small amount of spending money (perhaps small change or one-dollar bills) helps. If it is lost or given away, it is only a minimal amount. Sometimes a person needs to know that she has a little bit of cash on hand, and this is a way around conflicts about money. One peculiarity of the dementing diseases is that a person sometimes loses the ability to make change before she loses the knowledge that she needs money.

*Mrs. Hutchinson had always been fiercely independent about her money, so Mr. Hutchinson gave her a purse with some change in it. He put her name and address in it in case she lost her purse. She insisted on paying her hairdresser by check long after she could not responsibly manage a checkbook. So Mr. Hutchinson gave her some checks stamped VOID by the bank. Each week she gives one to the hairdresser. Mr. Hutchinson privately arranged with the hairdresser that these would be accepted and that he would pay the bills.*

This may seem extreme. It may also seem unfair to dupe the confused person this way. In reality this allows a sick woman to continue to feel independent and it allows her tired and burdened husband to manage the finances and keep the peace.

Money matters can cause serious problems, especially when the person is also suspicious or when other members of the family disagree. (It may be helpful here to read Chapters 8 and 11.) Your ingenuity can be a great help to you in making money matters less distressing.

## WHEN A PERSON CAN NO LONGER DRIVE SAFELY

The time may come when you realize that your parent or spouse can no longer drive safely. While some people will recognize their limits, others may be unwilling to give up driving.

For most experienced drivers, driving is a skill so well learned that it is partly "automatic." A person can go back and forth to work every day with her mind on other things—perhaps dictating or listening to music. It does not take much concentration to drive, but if the traffic pattern should suddenly change, she can rely on the mind to focus on the road immediately and respond swiftly to a crisis. Because driving is a well-learned skill, a confused person can still *appear* to be driving well when she is not really safe. Driving requires a highly complex interaction of eyes, brain, and muscle, and the ability to solve complicated problems quickly. A person who is still apparently driving safely may have lost the ability to respond appropriately to an unexpected problem on the road. She may be relying entirely on the habits of driving and may be unable to change quickly from a habitual response to a new response when the situation demands it.

Often people make the decision themselves to stop driving when they feel that they "aren't as sharp as they used to be." But if they do not, you have a responsibility to them and to others to assess carefully whether or not the person's driving is dangerous, and to intervene when it is. This may be one of the first situations in which you take a decision out of the hands of the impaired person. You may feel hesitant to do this, but you will probably be relieved once you have stopped a forgetful person from driving. To decide whether the time has come, look at the skills that a person needs to drive safely and evaluate whether the confused person still has these skills—both in the car and in other situations.

1. *Good vision:* A person must have good vision, or vision corrected with glasses, and be able to see clearly, both in front and out of the corners of her eyes (peripheral vision) so that she sees things coming toward her from the sides.

2. *Good hearing:* A person must be able to hear well or have her hearing corrected with a hearing aid, so that she is alert to the sounds of approaching cars, horns, and so forth.

3. *Quick reaction time:* A driver must be able to react quickly—to turn, to brake, and to avoid accidents. Older people's reaction time, when it is formally tested, is slightly slower than that of young people, but in well older people it is usually not slow enough to interfere with driving. However, if you see that a person seems slowed down or reacts slowly or inappropriately to sudden changes around the house, this should alert you to the possibility of the same limitations when she is driving.

4. *Ability to make decisions:* A driver must be able to make quick, *appropriate* decisions rapidly and *calmly*. The ability to make a correct decision when a child darts in front of the car, a horn honks, and a truck is approaching all at once necessitates being able to solve .complicated, unfamiliar problems quickly and without panicking. People with a dementing illness often rely on habitual responses that may not be the correct responses in a driving situation. Some people also get confused and upset when several things happen at once. You will see these problems, if they are occurring, around the house as well as in the car.

5. *Good coordination:* Eyes, hands, and feet must all still work together well to handle a car safely. If a person is getting clumsy, or if her way of walking has changed, it should alert you that she may also have trouble getting her foot on the brake.

6. *Alertness to what is going on around her:* A driver must be alert to all that is going on without becoming upset or confused. If a person is "missing things" that happen around her, she may no longer be a safe driver.

Sometimes driving behaviors alert you to problems. Forgetful people may get lost on routes that would not have confused them previously. Being lost can distract the driver and further interfere with her ability to react quickly. Sometimes driving too slowly is a clue that the driver is uncertain of her skills—but this does not mean that every cautious driver is an impaired driver.

Confused people may become angry or aggressive when they drive or they may inappropriately believe that other drivers are "out to get them." This is dangerous. Occasionally a person with a dementing illness is also drinking too much. Even small amounts of alcohol impair the driving ability of people with a brain injury. This is a dangerous combination, and you must intervene.

If you are concerned about a person's driving ability, you might first approach the problem by discussing it frankly with her. Even though a person is cognitively impaired she is still able to participate in decisions that involve her. How you initiate such a discussion may affect her response. People with brain impairments are sometimes less able to tolerate criticism than when they were well, so you will want to use tact in such a discussion. If you say, "Your driving is terrible, you are getting lost, and you're just not safe," a person may feel she has to defend herself and may argue with you. Instead, by gently saying, "You are getting absent-minded about stoplights," you may be able to give a person an "easy way out." Giving up driving can mean admitting one's increasing limitations. Look for ways to help the person save face and maintain her self-image at the same time you react to the need for safety. Try offering alternatives: "I'll drive today and you can look at the scenery." As a last resort some families have disconnected the battery or starter wire and told the impaired person that the car could not be repaired.

Sometimes a person will absolutely refuse to give up driving, despite your tact. It may help to enlist the support of the doctor or a family lawyer. Often a person will cooperate with the instructions of an authority when she may regard your advice as nagging. As a last resort you may have to take away the car keys. If you cannot do this, you can make it impossible to start a car by removing the distributor cap or the wire to the distributor. This is small and easy to replace when you want to drive. A gas station attendant can show you how to do this.

States vary in their policies regarding a driver's license. In some states the Department of Motor Vehicles will issue any nondriver an identification card that can be used to cash checks, etc. They will also investigate and sometimes suspend a license if they receive a written opinion from a physician that the person's health makes her an unsafe driver. Some states issue limited licenses that allow a person to drive only under certain circumstances, such as only in daylight. Call the state police or the Department of Motor Vehicles to find out the policy in your area.

## WHEN A PERSON CAN NO LONGER LIVE ALONE

When a person has lived alone but can no longer do so, the move to live with someone else can be difficult for everyone. Some people welcome the sense of security living with others provides. Others vigorously resist giving up their independence.

Often patients go through a series of stages from complete independence to living with someone. When a gradual transition from independence is possible, it may be easier for the person to adjust and it may postpone the time when she must live with someone. For example, at first the help of the neighbors or a Meals-on-Wheels program may be adequate; later, a family member or a paid helper may spend part of the day with the confused person. A person who is still fairly independent may only need someone to come in to give medications or help with a meal but not constant supervision.

Eventually, however, the time may come when the caregiving family decides that the person cannot live alone. You will need to be alert to the possibility that the person's ability to function alone can change suddenly: some minor stress or even a mild case of the flu can make her worse. Or, you may not notice the gradual, insidious decline until something happens. Here are some questions that will help you decide if that time has come.

Is the person eating her meals and taking her medications? A forgetful person may not eat, or may eat only sweets even when you have provided a hot meal. The person may take too much medicine or forget her medicine. This can make her mental impairment worse and can jeopardize her physical health. If the person is safe in other ways, she may be able to live alone if someone else helps daily with food and medicine, but it has been our experience that people who forget to eat properly are experiencing sufficient cognitive impairment that they probably cannot safely live alone.

Is the person able to manage her own personal care and grooming? Some forgetful people wear dirty clothes, forget (or refuse) to bathe or brush their teeth, or in other ways neglect themselves.

Is the person wandering away from home? She may get lost or be robbed or assaulted. Is the person wandering around outside at night? Such behavior is not uncommon and is dangerous.

Is the person forgetting to turn off the stove or burning the food? People who appear to be managing well often forget to turn off the stove. Is the person using candles or matches? It can be hard to believe that a person is really a danger to herself when she looks so well, but fire is a real and serious hazard. Cases of severe or even fatal accidental burns are not uncommon. If you suspect that the person is forgetting to turn off the stove, you must intervene.

Is the person keeping the house tidy, reasonably clean, and free of hazards? Forgetful people may spill puddles of water in the kitchen or bathroom and forget to clean them up. A person can slip and fall on a wet floor. Sometimes people forget to wash the dishes or forget to flush the toilet or in other ways create unsanitary conditions. If the house is badly cluttered, they can trip and fall. A confused person may pile up newspapers and rags which become a fire hazard.

Is the person keeping warm? A forgetful person may keep her house too cold or dress improperly. Her body temperature can drop dangerously if she does not keep herself warm. In hot weather the confused person may dress too warmly or may be afraid to open the house for adequate ventilation. This can lead to heat stroke.

Is the person acting in response to "paranoid" ideas or unrealistic suspiciousness? Such behavior can get her in trouble in the community. Sometimes people call the police because of their fears and make their neighbors angry. Sometimes, too, confused elderly people become the target of malicious teenagers. Such problems may occur in suburban neighborhoods as well in the inner city.

Is the person showing good judgment? Some confused people show poor judgment about whom they let in the house and can be robbed by the people they invite in, or they may give away money or do other inappropriate things.

## Moving to a New Residence

If some of these things are happening, you know that the person can no longer live alone and you must make other arrangements for her. You might consider full-time help or you may arrange for the person to move into someone else's home, a nursing home, or a sheltered housing setting. (These facilities will be described in detail in Chapter 16.)

*Mr. Sawyer reports, "Mother simply cannot live alone anymore. We hired a housekeeper and Mother fired her—and when I called the agency they said they could not send anyone else. So we talked with Mother, told her we wanted her to come live with us. But she absolutely refused. She says nothing is wrong with her, that I am trying to steal her money. She won't admit she isn't eating. She says she changed her clothes and we know she hasn't. I don't know what to do."*

If a confused person refuses to give up her independence and move into a safer setting, understanding something of what she may be thinking and feeling may help make the move easier. A move from independent living to living with someone else may mean giving up one's independence and admitting one's impairment. Moving means more losses. It means giving up a familiar place and often many familiar possessions. That place and those possessions are the tangible symbols of one's past and reminders when one's memories fail.

The confused person is dependent upon a familiar setting to provide her with cues that enable her to function independently. Learning one's way around in a new place is difficult or impossible. She feels dependent upon familiar surroundings to survive. The person with a dementing illness may forget the plans that have been discussed or may be unable to understand them. You may reassure your mother that she is coming to live in your house—which is very familiar to her—but all her damaged mind may perceive is that a lot of things are going to be lost.

As you make plans for this person to live with someone, there are several things to consider.

1. Take into careful consideration the changes that this move will mean in your life, and plan, before the move, for financial resources and emotional outlets and supports for yourself.

If the impaired person is to move in with you, what effect will this have on her income? Many states consider room and board as income and reduce Public Assistance benefits to people living with someone. You will also want to review such things as whether you can claim the person as your dependent on your income tax.

If the person is coming to live with you, how does the rest of the family feel about this? If there are children or teenagers in the family, will their activities upset the confused person or will the "odd" behavior of the confused person upset them? How does your spouse feel about this? Is your marriage already under stress? A demented person in the home creates burdens and stresses under the best of circumstances. If the demented person and her spouse are both moving in, you must also consider how the spouse will interact in the household. All of the people affected need to be involved in the decision and need the opportunity to express their concerns.

Assuming the care of a forgetful person may mean changes in other things: leisure time (you may not be able to go out because there is no one to sit with Mother), peace (you may not be able to read the newspaper or talk to your wife because Mother is pacing the floor), money (you may have increased medical bills, or bills for remodeling the bedroom), rest (the confused person may wake at night), visitors (people may stop visiting if the person's behavior is embarrassing). These are the things that make life tolerable and that help to reduce your stress. It is important to plan ways for you and your family to relax and get away from the problems of caring for a sick person. Remember also that other problems are not going to go away. You may still worry about your children, come home exhausted from your job, have the car break down, etc.

Is the person you are bringing into your home someone you can live with? If you never could get along with your mother and if her illness had made her behavior worse instead of better, having her move in with you may be disastrous. If you have had a long-standing poor relationship with the person who is now sick, that poor relationship is a reality that can make things more difficult for you.

2. Involve the person as much as possible in plans for the move, even if she refuses to move. The patient is still a person, and her participation in plans and decisions that involve her is important unless she is too severely impaired to comprehend what is happening. Confused people who have been hoodwinked into a move may become even more angry and suspicious and their adjustment to the new setting may be extremely difficult. Certainly the extent and nature of the impaired person's participation depend on the extent of her illness and her attitude toward the move.

Keep in mind that there is a key difference between making the decision, which you may have to do, and participating in the planning, which the confused person can be encouraged to do. Perhaps Mr. Sawyer's story will continue like this:

*"After we talked it over with Mother she still absolutely refused to consider a move. So I went ahead with the arrangements. I told Mother gently that she had to move because she was getting forgetful.*

*"I knew too many decisions at once would upset her, so we would just ask her a few things at a time. 'Mother, would*

*you like to take all your pictures with you?' 'Mother, let's take your own bed and your lovely bedspread for your new bedroom.'*

"Of course, we made a lot of decisions without her—about the stove and the washer, and the junk in the attic. And of course she kept saying she wasn't going and that I was robbing her. Still, I think some of it sank in, that she was 'helping' us get ready to move. Sometimes she would pick up a vase and say, 'I want Carol to have this.' We tried to comply with her wishes. Then after the move, we could honestly tell her that the vase was not stolen: she had given it to Carol."

When a person is too impaired to understand what is happening around her it may be better to make the move without the added stress of trying to involve her in it.

3. Be prepared for a period of adjustment. Changes are frequently upsetting to people with dementing illnesses. No matter how carefully and lovingly you plan the move, this is a major change, and the person may be upset for a while. It is easy to understand that it takes time to get over the losses a move involves. A forgetful person also needs extra time to learn her way around in a new place.

Reassure yourself that after an adjustment period the person usually will settle into her new surroundings. Signs on doors may help her find her way around an unfamiliar home. An additional sedative may help her sleep at night. Try to postpone other activities or changes until after everyone has adjusted to the move.

Occasionally an impaired person never really adjusts to moving. Don't blame yourself. You did the best you could and acted for her well-being. You may have to accept her inability to adjust as being the result of her illness.

# 5

## PROBLEMS ARISING IN DAILY CARE

### HAZARDS TO WATCH FOR

A PERSON WITH A DEMENTING ILLNESS is less able to take responsibility for his own safety. He is no longer able to evaluate consequences the way the rest of us do, and, because he forgets so quickly, accidents can easily happen. He may attempt to do familiar tasks without realizing that he can no longer manage them. For example, the disease may affect those portions of the brain which remember how to do simple things, such as buttoning buttons or slicing meat. This inability to do manual tasks is often unrecognized and causes accidents. Since the person also cannot learn, you will have to take special precautions to guard against accidents. Because a person seems to be managing well, you may not realize that he has lost the judgment he needs to avoid accidents. Families may need to take responsibility for the safety of even a mildly impaired person.

Accidents are most likely to occur when you are cross or tired, when everyone is hurrying, when there is an argument, or when someone in the household is sick. At these times you are less alert to the possibility of an accident and the impaired person may misunderstand or overreact to even the slightest mishap with a catastrophic reaction.

Do what you can to reduce confusion or tension when it arises. This is difficult when you are struggling with the care of a person with a dementing illness. If you are rushing with him to keep an appointment or finish a job, *stop*, even if it means being late or not getting something done. Catch your breath, rest a minute, and let the confused person calm down.

Be aware that mishaps can be warning signs of impending accidents: you banged your shin on the edge of the bed, or dropped and broke a cup, and the impaired person is getting upset. This is the time to create a change of pace before a serious accident occurs.

Alert others in the household to the relationship between increased tension and increased accidents. At such times everyone can keep a closer eye on the impaired person.

Be sure you know the limits of the impaired person's abilities. Do not take his word that he can heat up his supper or get into the tub alone. An occupational therapist can give you an excellent picture of what the person can do safely. If you do not have this resource, observe the person closely as he does various tasks.

Have an emergency plan ready in case something does happen. Whom will you call if someone is hurt? How will you get the upset person out in case of a fire? Remember that he may misinterpret what is happening and resist your efforts to help him.

Change the environment to make it safer. This is one of the most important ways to avoid accidents. Hospitals and other institutions have safety experts who regularly inspect for hazards. You can and should do the same thing. Go thoughtfully through your home, yard, neighborhood, and car, looking for things a person with a dementing illness could possibly misuse or misinterpret that might cause an accident.

## In the House

A neat house is safer than a cluttered one. There are fewer things to trip over or knock over, and hazards are more easily seen. Knickknacks or clutter may distract or confuse an impaired person.

Remove things that cause problems. If a person tries to use the iron and leaves it on, causing a fire hazard, put it away where he cannot find it. Whenever possible take the easiest path to safety without conflict. Does the impaired person have access to power tools, lawn mower, knives, hairdryer, stove, sewing machine, or car keys when he can no longer safely use them? You must put these in a locked closet.

Are all medications kept out of reach of a person who may forget that he has already taken them? Buy a metal file box from the dime store and equip it with an inexpensive lock to keep medications safely away from the forgetful person and visiting grandchildren.

Are things stored on the stairs? Clutter is always dangerous, particularly when a person is confused, clumsy, or misinterprets what he sees. Are extension cords stretched across the floor where a person might trip on them?

Lower the temperature on your water heater so that water is not hot enough to scald the person who accidentally turns it on. People with dementing illnesses can lose the ability to realize that hot water is too hot and they can burn themselves badly. Paint hot water taps bright red as a reminder. If hot water pipes are exposed, cover them with insulation.

If the confused person readjusts the furnace or water heater, you may need to lock the basement door.

If you have stairs, install gates at the top. The confused

person can easily get "turned around" and fall down the steps, especially at night. Check the handrails; be sure they are sturdy. Handrails should be anchored into the stud and not into drywall or plaster. They will not hold a person's weight if they are not securely fastened. Install handrails if there are none. As the person becomes unsteady on his feet, he will need them. Put away rugs that slip. If stairs are carpeted, check to see that the carpet is securely tacked down.

Remove furniture with sharp corners or sharp finials. Put away or block off large areas of breakable glass; a person can fall against a glass china cabinet and be badly cut. Put away rocking chairs that tip over easily. Put away coffee tables and fragile antiques.

Use stable chairs that are easy to get out of (see p. 52). Check to see if fingers or toes could get caught in parts of recliners. Furniture upholstery should be easy to clean; you may have to wipe up spills. Fabric, draperies, and cushions should be flame resistant.

Impaired people may not see well and it may become harder for them to distinguish colors that are similar to each other. Sometimes it helps to put bright reflector tape on handrails, doorways, and the corners of mantelpieces if a person has been bumping into them. (Also see Chapter 6: "Vision Problems.")

A confused person may fall out of a window. Lock windows securely. There are inexpensive devices to enable you to lock a window in an open position so that a person cannot get out but fresh air can get in. Open the window a little at the top and a little at the bottom and secure it.

Block off hot radiators by putting a sturdy chair in front of them. You may want to put a gate around a floor furnace.

Can the person lock himself in a room so that you cannot get in? Remove the lock, take the tumblers out, and replace the knob, or tape the latch open with tape.

Never keep insecticides, gasoline, paint, solvents, cleaning supplies, etc., in other than their original, clearly labeled containers. Store them safely out of reach of the confused person. Child-proof (and patient-proof) cabinet latches are available at hardware stores. Mildly confused people may try to use such materials inappropriately.

Impaired people forget what can be eaten and what cannot; they may drink solvents by mistake. These people may also eat other inappropriate items. Put small things such as pins and buttons out of reach. Give away poisonous houseplants. Some people will eat chips of loose paint from walls or furniture. Watch closely for any behavior that involves putting things in the mouth.

Most accidents happen in the kitchen and the bathroom. Confused people often try to turn on the stove but forget they have done so, or try to cook but put empty pans on a hot burner. *This is a serious fire hazard.* You must watch for this and intervene immediately. People left alone at home or those who get up at night are especially at risk.

You may be able to take the knobs off the stove so that the disabled person cannot operate it. If you have an electric stove, you can have a switch installed behind it so that when the switch is off the burners will not operate. You can remove the fuse or circuit breaker when you are not using the stove.

If you have a gas stove, ask the gas company to assist you in making the stove safe. Depending on the stove and your house, there are several things you can do. You may have to be quite persistent and talk to several people before you reach a company official who is helpful and understanding.

Confused people often spill water on the kitchen or bathroom floor and forget to wipe it up. It is easy to slip and fall on a wet spot, so watch for this and keep the floor dry. Perhaps you will want to give up waxing the floor, also. Waxing is work for you and makes the floor slippery.

Handrails and grab bars should be installed in the bathroom (see p. 99). They are available from medical supply houses.

Put a skid-resistant mat or decals on the floor of the tub or shower. It is sometimes helpful to replace the bathmat with bathroom carpeting. This is easily cleaned, doesn't slip, and soaks up puddles.

## Outdoors

Both adults and children can easily put a hand through the glass in a storm door. Storm doors should be covered with a protective grillwork. Sliding glass patio doors should be well marked with stick-on decals.

Check to see if a confused person might fall off a porch or deck. If there are steps, paint them bright, contrasting colors, attach outdoor no-skid tape to the edges, and install a banister.

Check for uneven ground, cracked pavement, holes in the lawn, fallen branches, thorny bushes, or molehills that the person can trip over.

Take down the clothesline so the person will not run into it.

Make sure the coals are out and cold on an outside barbecue. If you have a gas barbecue, be sure the confused person cannot operate it.

Lock up garden tools.

Check yard furniture to be sure it is stable, will not tip or collapse, and has no splinters or chipped paint.

Fence in or dispose of poisonous flowers.

*Outdoor swimming pools are very dangerous.* Be sure that yours or your neighbor's is securely fenced and locked so that the person cannot get to it. You may have to explain carefully the nature of the person's disability to the owner of a pool, making certain that the confused person is not ever assumed to be competent around a pool. Even if he has always been a good swimmer, a confused person may lose his judgment or his ability to handle himself in the water.

## In the Car

Problems with driving are discussed in Chapter 4. Never leave a confused person alone in a car. He may wander away, fiddle with the ignition, release the handbrake, be harassed by strangers, or run the battery down with the lights. Automatic windows are dangerous for confused people and for children, who may close the window on their head or arm.

Occasionally a confused person will open the car door and attempt to get out while the car is moving. Locking the doors may help. If this continues to be a problem, you may need a third person to drive while you keep the impaired person calm. In some cases you can unscrew and remove the knobs on the door locks so that the person cannot unlock the door while you are driving.

## Smoking

If the person smokes, the time will come when he lays lighted cigarettes down and forgets them. *This is a serious hazard.* If it occurs, you must intervene. Try to discourage smoking. Many families have taken cigarettes completely away from a patient. Things may be difficult for a few days or weeks, but much easier in the long run.

Other families allow the impaired person to smoke only under their supervision. All smoking materials and matches must be kept out of reach of the forgetful person. (The person who has cigarettes but no matches may use the stove to light his cigarette and may leave the stove on.)

## NUTRITION AND MEALTIMES

Good nutrition is important to both you and the chronically ill person. If you are not eating well, you will be more tense and more easily upset. It is not known to what extent a proper diet affects the progress of dementing diseases, but we do know that forgetful people often fail to eat properly and can suffer nutritional deficiencies. Sometimes this can make symptoms worse.

A balanced daily diet as recommended by the Council on Foods and Nutrition of the American Medical Association includes: two or more glasses of milk (or cheese, ice cream, or cottage cheese); two or more servings of meat, fish, poultry, eggs, cheese, or dry beans, peas, or nuts; four or more servings of vegetables and fruits, including dark green or yellow vegetables, citrus fruit, or tomatoes; and four or more servings of enriched or whole-grain breads and cereals. Both you and the person with a dementing illness need this balanced diet to avoid other illnesses and to cope with the stress of a chronic illness. If your doctor has recommended a special diet for managing other diseases like diabetes or heart disease, it is important that you know from him what foods you should eat in order to maintain a balanced diet. He can refer you to a nutritionist or a nurse who can help you manage a special diet.

There is no known link between nutrition and Alzheimer's disease and there are no special diets that have proven to help memory problems.


## Meal Preparation

When you must prepare meals on top of all your other responsibilities you may find yourself taking short cuts such as fixing just a cup of coffee and toast for yourself and the confused person. If preparing meals is a job you had to take on for the first time when your spouse became ill, you may not know how to serve good nutritious meals quickly and easily and you may not want to learn to cook. There are several alternatives. We suggest you plan a variety of ways to get good meals with a minimum of effort.

There are Eating Together programs for people over sixty and Meals-on-Wheels programs in most areas. Both services provide one hot, nutritious meal a day. You can find out what meal services are available through a social worker or by calling the local office on aging. Meals-on-Wheels programs bring a meal to your home. Eating Together programs, funded under the Older Americans Act, provide lunch and often a recreation program in the company of other retired people at a community center. Transportation is often provided.

Many restaurants will prepare carry-out meals if requested. This helps when a person can no longer eat in public.

There are numerous inexpensive cookbooks on the market that explain the basic steps in easy meal preparation. Some are written for the man who is "bacheloring." Some are in large print. An experienced homemaker can show you how to prepare quick, easy meals. The home economist in your county extension office or the public health nurse can give you good, easy recipes for two. She also has helpful information on budgeting, shopping, meal planning, and nutrition, and she can help you understand and plan menus for special diets.

Use TV dinners only as an emergency back-up. They are not an adequate regular diet. They are low in vitamins, high in salt, and lack the roughage older people need to prevent constipation.

## Problem Eating Behaviors

Forgetful people who are still eating some meals alone may forget to eat, even if you leave food in plain sight. They may hide food, throw food away, or eat it after it has spoiled. These are signals that the person can no longer manage alone and that you must make new arrangements. You may manage for a time by phoning at noon to remind him to eat lunch now, but this is a short-term solution. Confused people who live alone are frequently malnourished. Even when they appear overweight, they may not be getting the proper foods.

Many of the problems that arise at mealtime involve catastrophic reactions. Make mealtime as regular a routine as possible, with as little confusion as you can arrange. This will help prevent catastrophic reactions. Fussy or messy eaters do better when things are calm.

Check that dentures are tight fitting if the person uses them to eat. If they are loose, it may be safer to leave them out until they can be adjusted.

Check the temperature of foods, especially food heated in a microwave oven. Confused people often lack the judgment to avoid burning themselves.

People with dementing illnesses may develop rigid likes and dislikes and refuse to eat certain foods. Such people may be more willing to eat familiar foods, prepared in familiar ways. If the person never liked a particular food, he will not like it now. New foods may confuse him. If the person insists on eating only one or two things and if all efforts at persuasion or disguising foods fail, you will need to ask the doctor about vitamins and diet supplements.

If the person has a complicating illness, such as diabetes, which requires a special diet, it may be necessary to put foods he should not eat where he cannot get them, and allow him only those foods he should have. Remember, he may lack the judgment to decide responsibly between his craving and his well-being. Since a proper diet is important to his health, you may have to be responsible for preventing him from getting foods he should not have, even if he vigorously objects. A locksmith can put a lock on the refrigerator door if necessary. Childproof locks will secure cabinets. But before you invest in locks, ask yourself whether you need to keep all those sweets around anyway.

People with dementing illnesses may be unable to recognize that some things are not good to eat. You may need to lock up foods like salt, vinegar, oil, or Worcestershire sauce, which can make the person sick if he eats them in quantity.

### Nibbling

Sometimes a person seems to forget that he ate, and will ask for food again right after a meal. Sometimes people seem to want to eat all the time. Try setting out a tray of small, nutritious "nibbles" such as small crackers or cheese cubes. Sometimes people will take one at a time and be satisfied. If weight gain is a problem, put out carrots or celery.

### Messiness

If the person has problems with coordination he may lose the ability to do tasks he has always done. When this happens, he may become a messy eater, and may begin using his fingers instead of silverware or begin to spill food. It is usually easier to adjust to this than to fight circumstances.

Use a plastic tablecloth or plastic placemats. Try a clear plastic cloth over a pretty tablecloth. Get the person an attractive smock to wear, rather than a bib, if spills are a problem. Turn the bottom up into a big pocket to catch crumbs. Variety stores sell the large plastic smock used by beauticians. This makes an excellent apron.

Put only the utensil (fork or spoon) that the person will need at his place. Utensils with large, built-up handles are easier for people with poor coordination. You can purchase these or build up your own handle with foam rubber. A fork or spoon with some weight will help the person remember that he is holding it. Forgetful people may not remember that they are holding plastic forks or they may bite off pieces of them.

In general, it is easier for a person to manage a bowl than a plate. Use sturdy plastic rather than glass or china dishes. Use dishes that are a different color from the placemat. Glass is hard to see. To keep a plate from sliding, place Dycem, a nylon material sold in medical supply houses, under the plate or attach suction cups to the bottom of the plate. Plates with suction cups are available from medical supply companies and are also sold for children. If neither is available, a damp washcloth under the plate will help keep it from sliding. To keep food from being pushed off a dish, a plate guard can be temporarily attached to any plate or you can use a scoop dish. Both are available from medical supply houses.

Some people lose the ability to judge how much liquid will fill a glass and overfill glasses. They will need your help. If a person dribbles or spills when drinking from a cup, use a convalescent feeding cup, which has a plastic cover with a spout. Similar spillproof cups are also sold for children. Don't fill glasses or cups full. This will help prevent spilling.

As eating becomes more difficult, limit the number of foods you put in front of the confused person at one time. For example, serve only his salad, then only his meat. Having to make choices is often what leads to playing in the food. Don't put salt, ketchup, etc., where he can reach it and mix it inappropriately into his food. Season his food for him. Be sure that food is cut into pieces that are small and tender enough to be eaten safely. People with dementing illnesses may forget to chew or fail to cut meats up properly, because the hands and brain no longer work together.

If you spoonfeed a person, put only a small amount of food on the spoon at a time, and wait until the person swallows before giving him the next bite. You may have to remind him verbally to swallow.

## Fluids

Be sure that the person gets enough fluid each day. Even mildly impaired people may forget to drink, and inadequate fluids can lead to other physical problems. (See p. 113.)

Don't give the person a cup of tea or coffee that is too hot to drink. He will eventually lose the ability to judge this and will burn himself.

### Puréed Diet

If the person is on a puréed diet, use a babyfood grinder. You can purée normally prepared foods in it. This saves time and money. Home-cooked foods will be more appealing to the person than babyfoods.

### Drooling or Respiratory Problems

If the person drools or has respiratory problems, milk or citrus juice may produce more mucus and make the problem worse. Check with your doctor to determine the cause of the problem. Then offer fruit nectar or cranberry juice instead of orange juice or milk.

## Weight Loss

Sometimes a person with a severe dementia stops eating. This can be a difficult and frustrating situation. If a person stops eating or begins to lose weight, notify the doctor. This can be a signal of a complicating disease. It is important to search carefully for any contributory physical illness. Is the person depressed? Does he have an acute illness (see p. 110)? Has he had a stroke? Be sure to check for painful teeth or gums or poorly fitting dentures.

Sometimes a familiar person can coax a patient to eat. Offer his favorite foods. If they must be puréed, be sure they are still tasty. Put only one thing on his plate at a time. Often an impaired person eats slowly. Be sure he is not rushed. Be sure that his physical surroundings are pleasant, calm, and not distracting. We have had one patient respond by having her back gently stroked while she was being fed. One patient responded to a low dose of neuroleptic given one hour before meals.

You may give a person who is not eating well a liquid high-calorie diet supplement like Ensure or Mariteme. You can purchase these by the case from most pharmacies. They contain the vitamins, minerals, and proteins the person needs. They come in different flavors; the person may like some better than others. Offer this as the beverage with a meal or as a "milk shake" between meals. Consult your physician.

If all efforts fail and the person continues to refuse to eat, you and the doctors are left with an ethical dilemma. Should you feed the patient through a nasogastric (NG) tube (a tube that goes through the nose into the stomach)? Should you insert a feeding tube directly into the stomach? Or should you allow the patient to die? Only you can make these decisions.

## Choking

Sometimes people with coordination problems begin to have trouble swallowing. If the person has difficulty changing his facial expression, he may also have trouble chewing or swallowing. When this occurs, it is important to guard against choking. Do not give the person foods that he may forget to chew thoroughly, such as small hard candy, nuts, carrots, chewing gum, or popcorn. Soft, thick foods are less likely to cause choking. Easy to handle foods include chopped meat, soft-boiled eggs, canned fruit, and frozen yogurt. Foods can be ground in a blender. Seasoning will make them more appealing.

If the person has trouble swallowing, be sure he is sitting up straight with his head slightly forward—never tilted back when he eats. He should be sitting in the same position in which a well person would sit at a table. He should remain sitting for fifteen minutes after he eats.

Do not feed a person who is agitated or sleepy.

Foods like milk and cereal may cause choking. The two textures—liquid and solid—make it hard for him to know whether to chew or swallow.

Some fluids are easier to swallow than others. If a person tends to choke on fluids like water, try a thicker liquid. A nurse can help you cope with this problem.

## First Aid for Choking

A nurse or the Red Cross can teach you a very simple technique that can save the life of a choking person. It takes only a few minutes to learn this simple skill. Everyone should know how to do it.

If the person can talk, cough, or breathe, *do not interfere*. If the person cannot talk, cough, or breathe (and he may point to his throat or turn bluish), *you must help him*. If he is in a chair or standing, stand behind him, then reach around him and lock or overlap your two hands in the middle of his abdomen (belly) below the ribs. Pull hard and quickly back and up (toward you). If he is lying down, turn him so he is face up, put your two hands in the middle of his belly, and push. This will force air up through the throat and cause the food to fly out like a cork out of a bottle. (You can practice where to put your hands, but you should not push hard on a breathing person.)

## EXERCISE

Remaining physically fit is an important part of good health. We do not know the precise role that exercise plays in good health, but we do know that it is important for both you and the confused person to get enough exercise. Perhaps exercise will refresh you after the daily burdens of caring for a chronically ill person. We do not know the relationship between tension and exercise, but many people who lead intense, demanding lives are convinced that physical exercise enables them to handle pressure more effectively.

Dementia is not caused by inadequate circulation. Therefore, improving circulation with exercise does not prevent or reverse memory disorders, but it does have other useful effects.

Some practitioners have observed that people with dementing illnesses who exercise regularly seem to be calmer and do less agitated pacing. Some have observed that motor skills seem to be retained longer if they are used regularly. Exercise is a good way to keep an impaired person involved in activities, since it may be easier for him to use his body than to think and remember. Perhaps of most importance to you is the fact that sufficient exercise seems to help confused people sleep at night, and it helps to keep their bowel movements regular.

You may have to exercise with the impaired person. The kind of exercise you do depends on what you and the impaired person enjoy. There is no point to adding an odious exercise program to your life. Consider what the person did before he got sick and find ways to modify that activity so that it can continue. Sometimes an exercise project can also be a time for you and the impaired person to share closeness and affection without having to talk.

How much exercise can an older person safely do? If you or the impaired person has high blood pressure or a heart condition, check with the doctor before you do anything. If both of you can do normal walking around the house, climb steps, and shop for groceries, you can do a moderate exercise program. Always start a new activity gradually and build up slowly. If an exercise causes either of you stiffness, pain, or swelling, do less of it or change to a gentler activity. Check the person's feet for blisters or bruises if you begin walking.

## Simple Exercises

Walking is excellent exercise. Try to take the person outside for a short walk in all but the worst weather. The movement and the fresh air may help him sleep better. If the weather is too rainy or cold, drive to a shopping mall. Make a game of "window shopping." Be sure both of you have comfortable, low-heeled shoes, and soft, absorbent cotton socks. You may gradually build up the distance you walk, but avoid steep hills. It may be easier for a forgetful person to walk the same route each day. Point out scenery, people, smells, etc., as you walk.

Dancing is good exercise. If the person enjoyed dancing before he became ill, encourage some sort of movements to music.

If the person played golf or tennis, he may be able to enjoy hitting the ball around long after he became unable to play a real game.

Confused people often enjoy doing calisthenics as part of a group, for example, in a day care setting. If you are doing exercises in a group or at home, try having him imitate what you are doing. If he has trouble with specific movements, try gently helping him move.

If the person is able to keep his balance, standing exercises are better than those done sitting in a chair. However, if balance is a problem, do the same exercises from a chair.

Even people who are confined to bed can exercise. However, exercises for seriously chronically ill patients must be planned by a physical therapist so they do not aggravate other conditions and are not dangerous to a person who has poor coordination or poor balance.

Exercise should be done at the same time each day, in a quiet, orderly way, so it does not create confusion that would add to the person's agitation. Follow the same sequence of exercises, starting from the head and working your way down toward the feet. Make the exercises fun and encourage the person to remember them. If the person has a catastrophic reaction, stop and try again later.

The impaired person may have other physical problems that

interfere with his ability to exercise. You should notify your doctor of any new physical problems and of marked changes in existing ones.

When a person has been sick or inactive, he may become weak and tire more easily. He may get stiff joints. Regular, gentle exercise can help keep his joints and his muscles in healthy condition. When stiffness or weakness is caused by other diseases such as arthritis or by injury, a physical or occupational therapist can plan an exercise program that may help prevent further stiffness or weakness.

## RECREATION

Recreation, having fun, and enjoying life are important for everyone. A dementing illness does not mean an end to enjoying life. It may mean that you will need to make a special effort to find things that give pleasure to the impaired person. Previously enjoyed activities may remain important and enjoyable even for seriously impaired people. However, the things the person used to enjoy, such as hobbies, guests, concerts, or going out to dinner, can become too complicated to be fun for someone who is easily confused. These must be replaced by simpler joys, although it can be hard for family members to understand that simple things can now give just as much pleasure.

Music is a delightful resource for many confused people. Sometimes a severely impaired person seems to retain a capacity to enjoy old, familiar songs. He may be able to use a simple tape deck or radio with large knobs. Very impaired people are sometimes still able to play the piano or sing if they learned this skill earlier.

Some memory-impaired people enjoy television. Others get upset when they cannot understand the story any more. The quick shifts from one scene to another precipitate catastrophic reactions in some people.

Most confused people enjoy seeing old friends, although sometimes visitors upset them. If this happens, try having only one or two people visit at a time, instead of a group. It is often the confusion of several people at once that is upsetting. Ask visitors to stay for shorter periods, and explain to them the reason for the person's forgetfulness and other behaviors.

Some families enjoy going out to dinner, and many people with dementing illnesses retain their social graces well. Others embarrass the family by their messy eating. It is helpful to order for the confused person and select simple foods that can be eaten neatly. Remove unnecessary glasses and silverware. Some families have found that it helps to explain to the waitress discreetly that the person is confused and cannot order for himself.

Consider the hobbies and interests the person had before he became ill, and look for ways he can still enjoy these. Often, for example, people who liked to read continue to enjoy leafing through magazines after they can no longer make sense of the text. Sometimes a person puts away a hobby or interest and refuses to pick it up again. This often happens with something a person had done well and can no longer do as effectively. It can seem degrading to encourage a person to do a simplified version of a once fine skill unless he particularly enjoys it. It may be better to find new kinds of recreation.

Everyone enjoys experiencing things through his senses. You probably enjoy watching a brilliant sunset, smelling a flower, or tasting your favorite food. People with dementia are often more isolated and may not be able to seek out experiences to stimulate their senses. Try pointing out a pretty picture, a bird singing, a familiar smell or taste. Remember the sense of touch. The person may enjoy stroking a furry animal, touching a smooth piece of wood, or putting his hand under running water. Like you, the person will enjoy certain sensations more and others less.

Many families have found that confused people enjoy a ride in the car.

If the person has always enjoyed animals, he may respond with delight to pets. Some cats and dogs seem to have an instinctive way with brain-impaired people.

As the dementing illness continues and the person develops trouble with coordination and language, it is easy to forget his need to experience pleasant things and to enjoy himself.

Never overlook the importance of hand holding, touching, hugging, and loving. Often when there is no other way we can find to communicate with a person, he will respond to touching. Touch is an important part of human communication. You may enjoy just sitting and holding hands. It's a good way to share some time when talking has become difficult or impossible.

## Meaningful Activity

Much of what a well person does during the day has a purpose that gives meaning and importance to life. We work to make money, to serve others, to feel important. We may knit a sweater for a grandchild, or bake a cake for a friend. We wash our hair and clothes so we will look nice and be clean. Such purposeful activities are important to us—they make us feel useful and needed.

When the person with a dementing illness is unable to continue his usual activities, you need to help him find things to do that are meaningful and still within his abilities. Such tasks should be meaningful and satisfying to him—whether they seem so to you or not. A man may be able to spade a garden for you and for the neighbors. A woman may be able to peel the vegetables or set the table when she is no longer able to prepare a complete meal. Confused people can wind a ball of yarn, dust, or stack magazines while you do the housework. Encourage the person to do as much as he can for himself, although you can simplify the tasks for him.

## PERSONAL HYGIENE

The amount of help a person with a dementing illness needs in personal care varies with the extent of his brain damage. The person with Alzheimer's disease will be able to care for himself in the early stages of the disease, but may gradually begin to neglect himself and will eventually need total help.

Problems often arise over getting a person to change his clothes or take a bath. "I already changed," the person may tell you, or he may turn the tables and make it sound as if you are wrong to suggest such a thing.

*A daughter says, "I can't get her to change clothes. She has had the same clothes on for a week. She sleeps in them. When I tell her to change, she says she already did or she yells at me, 'Who do you think you are, telling me when to change my clothes?'"*

*A husband relates, "She screams for help the whole time I am bathing her. She'll open the windows and yell, 'Help, I'm being robbed.'"*

A person with a dementing illness may become depressed or apathetic and lose any desire to clean up. He may be losing the ability to remember how much time has passed: it doesn't *seem* like a week since he changed clothes. To have someone telling him he needs to change his clothes may embarrass him. (If someone came up to you and told you that you should change your clothes, you might well become indignant.)

Dressing and bathing are personal activities. We each have our own individual ways of doing things. Some of us take showers, some take tub baths, some of us bathe in the morning, some bathe at night. Some of us change clothes twice a day, some every other day, but each of us is quite set in our way of doing things. Sometimes when a family member begins to help the demented person, he inadvertently overlooks these established habits. The change in routine can be upsetting to the confused person. A generation ago, people often did not wash and change as often as we do today. Once a week may have been the way the person did things in his childhood.

We begin to bathe and dress ourselves as small children. It is a basic indication of our independence. Moreover, bathing and dressing are private activities. Many people have never completely bathed and dressed in front of anyone else. Having other people's hands and eyes on our naked, aging, not-so-beautiful body is an acutely uncomfortable experience. When we offer to help with something a person has always done for himself—something everybody does for himself and does in private—it is a strong statement that this person is not able to do for himself any longer, that he has, in fact, become like a child who must be told when to dress and must have help.

Changing clothes and bathing involve making many decisions. A man must select among many socks, shirts, and ties for an outfit that goes together. When he begins to realize he can't do this, when looking at a drawer full of blue, green, and black socks becomes overwhelmingly confusing, it can be easier just not to change.

Such factors as these often precipitate catastrophic reactions involving bathing and dressing. Still, you are faced with the problem of keeping this person clean. Begin by trying to understand the person's feelings and his need for privacy and independence. Know that his behavior is a product of his brain impairment, and is not deliberately offensive. Look for ways to simplify the number of decisions involved in bathing and dressing without taking away his independence.

## Bathing

When a person refuses to take a bath, part of the problem may be that the business of bathing has become too confusing and complicated. Try to follow as many of the person's old routines as possible while you encourage him to bathe, and at the same time simplify the job for him. If a man has always shaved first, then showered, then eaten breakfast, he is most likely to cooperate with your request if you time it for before breakfast. Then lay out his clothes and towels and start the water.

Be calm and gentle when you help with a bath. Avoid getting into discussions about whether a bath is needed. Instead, tell the person *one step at a time* what to do in preparation for the bath.

Avoid: *"Dad, I want you to take a bath right after breakfast."* (*"Right after breakfast"* means he has to remember something.)

Avoid: *"I don't need a bath."* *"Oh yes you do. You haven't had a bath in a week."* (You would not like him saying that to you, especially if you couldn't remember when you last had a bath.)

Try: *"Dad, your bath water is ready."* *"I don't need a bath."* *"Here is your towel. Now, unbutton your shirt."* (His mind may focus on the buttons instead of on the argument. You can gently help him if you see him having difficulty.) *"Now stand up. Undo your pants, Dad."* *"I don't need a bath."* *"Now step into the tub."*

The bath should be a regular routine, done the same way at the same time. The person will come to expect this and may put up less resistance. When bathing continues to be difficult, it is not necessary for the person to bathe every day. Always check the temperature of the bath or shower water, even if the person has been successfully doing this for himself. The ability to gauge safe temperatures can be lost quite suddenly. Avoid using bubble bath or bath oils that can make the tub slippery. These can also contribute to vaginal infections in women.

Showers are more dangerous than tub baths because the unsteady person may fall. If you must use a shower, install grab bars or use a tub seat. There are several inexpensive appliances that you can rent or purchase that make bathing much safer and easier (see p. 98).

Never leave the person alone in the tub. Use only two or three inches of water. This helps the person feel more secure, and is safer in case he slips. Put a rubber mat or no-skid decals on the bottom of the tub. People can often continue to wash themselves if you gently remind them one step at a time of each area to wash.

Sometimes it is embarrassing for a family member to see that the genital area is thoroughly washed, but rashes can develop, so see that this is done. Be sure that you or the confused person has washed in folds of flesh and under breasts.

Use a bathmat that will not slip for the person to step out onto and be sure there are no puddles on the floor. It may be helpful to replace bathmats with bathroom carpeting that does not slip, soaks up puddles, and is washable. If the person still dries himself, check to see that he doesn't forget some areas. If you dry the person, be sure he is completely dry. Use body powder, baby powder, or cornstarch under women's breasts and in creases and folds of skin. Cornstarch is an inexpensive, odorless, and nonallergenic substitute for talcum powder. Baking soda is an effective substitute if the person resists using a deodorant.

While the person is undressed, check for red areas of skin, rashes, or sores. If any red areas or sores appear, ask your physician to help you manage them. Pressure sores or decubitus ulcers develop quickly on people who sit or lie down much of the time. Use body lotion on dry skin. There are unscented lotions for men.

## Dressing

If all of the person's socks will go with all of his slacks, he doesn't have to decide which is right to wear with what.

Hang ties, scarves, or accessories on the hanger with the shirt or dress they go with. Eliminate belts, scarves, sweaters, ties, and other accessories that are likely to be put on wrong.

Lay out a clean outfit for the confused person. Laying out clothes in the order in which he puts them on may also help.

Put away out-of-season or rarely worn clothes so they do not add to the decisions the person must make. If the person refuses to change clothes, avoid getting in an argument. Make the suggestion again later.

As the disease progresses, it becomes difficult for a person to get clothes on right side out and in the right sequence. Buttons, zippers, shoe laces, and belt buckles become impossible to manage. If the person can no longer manage buttons, replace them with Velcro tape, which you can purchase in a fabric store. People can often manage this after their fingers can no longer cope with buttons. One wife, sensitive to her husband's need to continue to dress himself independently, bought him clothes that were reversible. She bought attractive t-shirts, which don't look bad if they are worn backward and which don't have buttons, pants with elastic waistbands, and tube socks. (Tube socks don't have heels, so it takes less skill to put them on.) Slip-on shoes are easier than shoes with laces or ties.

Women can look pretty in reversible, slip-on blouses and reversible, wrap-around or elastic-waistband skirts or slacks. Loose-fitting clothing is easier to manage.

Select clothing that is washable and that doesn't need ironing; there is no reason to add to your work load.

Sometimes bright, "busy" patterns confuse and distract the impaired person. Try simpler patterns and pastel colors. Select colors with considerable contrast; these are easier for the older person to distinguish.

Women's underwear is difficult for a confused person to manage, and a mystery to many husbands. Buy soft, loose-fitting panties. It won't matter if they are on backward or wrong side out. Skip the slip; it is not necessary. If you must put a bra on a woman, ask her to lean forward to settle her breasts in the cups. Pantyhose are difficult to put on, and knee socks or garter belts are bad for people with poor circulation. Short cotton socks may be best to wear at home.

## Grooming

Have the person's hair cut in an atrractive, short style that is easy to wash and care for. Avoid a style that requires setting. People who have always gone to the beauty shop or barber shop may still enjoy doing so. If this is too upsetting an experience, it may be possible to arrange for a beautician or barber to come to your home.

It may be safer (and easier on your back) to wash hair in the kitchen sink rather than the tub unless you have a sprayer attached to the bathtub. Invest in a hose attachment for the sink. Be sure you rinse hair well. It should squeak when rubbed through your fingers.

You will need to trim fingernails and toenails or check to see that he can still do this.

Encourage the person to get dressed and to look nice. Moping around in a bathrobe will not help his morale. If a woman has always worn makeup it may be good for her to help her continue to wear simple makeup. It is not difficult for a husband to put powder and lipstick on his wife. Use pastel colors and a light touch on an older woman. Skip the eye makeup.

When the bath and dressing are finished, encourage the person to look in the mirror and see how nice he looks (even if you are exhausted and exasperated). Get the rest of the family to compliment him also. Praise and encouragement are important in helping him continue to feel good about himself even when a task he has always been able to do, such as dressing, has become too much for him.

## Oral Hygiene

With all the other chores of caring for a chronically ill person it is easy to forget what we can't see, but good oral hygiene is important for the person's comfort and for his health. A person who appears to be able to care for himself in other ways may, in fact, be forgetting to care for his teeth or dentures.

Dentures are particularly troublesome. If they don't fit just right or if a person is not applying the denture adhesive properly, they interfere with chewing. The natural response is to stop eating those things one can't chew. This can lead to inadequate nutrition or constipation. Dentures should be in place when a person is eating. If they don't fit properly or are uncomfortable, insist that the dentist fix them. If a person forgets to take his dentures out and clean them, or if he refuses to let you do it, he can develop painful sores on his gums which also interfere with a proper diet.

Since you want the person to be as independent as possible, you can assume the responsibility of remembering, but let the person do as much of the actual care as possible. One reason people stop caring for their teeth or dentures is that these are actually complicated tasks with many steps and they get confused about what to do next. You can help by breaking down the job into simple steps and reminding the person one step at a time. If you take over the care of the person's dentures, you must remove them daily, clean them, and check the gums for irritation. The dentist can show you how to do this. If the person has his own teeth, you may have to brush them for him and check the mouth for sores. Make oral care a part of a regular, expected routine and do it calmly; you will get less resistance. Select a time of day when the person is most cooperative. If the person does get upset, stop, and try again later.

Healthy teeth or properly fitting dentures are critically important. People with dementing illnesses tend not to chew well and to choke easily. Poor teeth make this worse. Even mild nutritional problems caused by sore teeth can increase the person's confusion or cause constipation. Sores in the mouth can lead to other problems and can increase the person's impairment.

## Bathroom Supplies

Medical supply houses carry a variety of bathroom aids which make the bathroom safer and easier for the impaired person.

Raised toilet seats make it easier for an impaired person to get off and on the seat and easier to transfer a person from a wheelchair to the toilet. The seat should fasten securely to the toilet so it does not slip when the person sits on it. Padded (soft) toilet seats are more comfortable for the person who must sit for some time. This is especially important for the person who develops pressure sores easily. At least one manufacturer sells a raised, padded seat.

You can rent portable commodes that can be placed near a person's bed or on the ground floor, so that the person does not have to climb stairs. Urinals and bedpans are available to meet a variety of needs. Discuss your specific problem with the supply house so that they can help you select the appliance that is best for you.

Grab bars are important. There are bars that help a person lift himself off and on the toilet and bars that he can grasp as he gets in and out of the bathtub. You can rent or buy bars that mount into your wall (and the rental agency may install them for you) or that are free standing or clamp onto the tub. These latter are helpful if you are renting your home and cannot attach things to the walls.

Towel racks and the bar on the soap dish in many homes and apartments are glued to the wall or fastened only into the wallboard. They may come loose if a person grabs them for balance or to lift himself up. Ask someone knowledgeable about carpentry to be sure they are anchored into the stud in the wall or are designed for the purpose. A seat for the shower or tub can be purchased or rented. This often makes a person feel more secure and raises him up so that you can reach him without so much bending and stretching. Hose attachments are helpful for rinsing the person thoroughly and they make washing hair much easier.

Grab bars, bath seats, and hoses are sold and rented by medical supply houses, large drug stores, and some department stores. They come in a variety of different designs to fit different bathrooms and to meet different needs. Medicare, Medicaid, or major medical insurance may pay part or all of the rental cost of equipment ordered by a physician.

## INCONTINENCE (WETTING OR SOILING)

People with dementing illnesses may begin to wet themselves or have their bowel movements in their clothing. This is called, respectively, urinary incontinence and bowel or fecal incontinence. The two are really separate problems, and one often occurs without the other. There are many causes of incontinence, so it is important to begin by assessing the problem.

Urinating and moving one's bowels are natural human

functions. However, ever since childhood we have been taught that these are private activities. Many of us have also been taught that they are nasty, dirty, or socially unacceptable. In addition, we associate caring for our own body functions in private with independence and personal dignity. When another person has to help us, it is distressing for both the helper and the disabled person. Often, too, people find urine or bowel movements disgusting and may gag or vomit when cleaning up. It is important for both family members and professional care givers to be aware of their own strong feelings in these areas.

## Urinary Incontinence

Urinary incontinence has many causes, some of which respond well to treatment. Ask yourself the following questions.

If the person is a woman, is she "leaking" rather than completely emptying her bladder, especially when she laughs, coughs, lifts something, or makes some other sudden exertion? Do accidents happen only at certain times of day, such as at night? (It is helpful to keep a diary for several days of the times accidents occur, the times the person successfully uses the toilet, and the times the person eats or drinks.) How often does the person urinate? Is the urination painful? Did the incontinence begin suddenly? Has the person's confusion suddenly gotten worse? Does the incontinence occur occasionally or intermittently? Is the person living in a new place? Is the person urinating in improper places, such as in closets or in flower pots? (This is different from the person who wets himself and his clothing wherever he happens to be.) Do accidents happen when the person cannot get to the bathroom on time? Are they happening on the way to the bathroom?

Whenever incontinence begins, it is important to check with the doctor. You can help him diagnose the problems by having the answers to these questions. If the person has a fever, report this to the doctor at once.

Incontinence may be brought on by either chronic or acute bladder infections, uncontrolled diabetes, a fecal impaction, an enlarged prostate, dehydration, medications, or many other medical problems. (See Chapter 6: "Medical Problems.") Do not let a physician dismiss incontinence without carefully exploring all possible treatable causes.

"Leaking" can be caused by weakening muscles and other conditions that are potentially treatable.

If the problem is that the person who moves slowly or uses a walker or who is clumsy cannot get to the bathroom in time, you can bring the toilet closer to the person. For example, if a person must go upstairs to the toilet, renting a commode for the ground floor may solve the problem. You can improvise a portable urinal that will help when you travel. You can also simplify clothing so the awkward person can manipulate it faster. Try Velcro tape instead of zippers or buttons. Can the person easily get up out of his chair? If he is sunk in a deep chair, he may not be able to get up in time.

Sometimes people cannot find the bathroom. This often happens in a new setting. A clear sign or a brightly painted door may help. People who urinate in wastebaskets, closets, and flowerpots may be unable to locate the bathroom or unable to remember the appropriate place. Some families find that putting a lid on the waste basket, locking closet doors, and taking the person to the bathroom on a regular schedule help. Remember that older people may have been taught as children to urinate outdoors or in a can by the bed. If so, it may be easier to supply them with a can than to clean up the waste basket.

Purchase washable chair cushion covers. Slide them on over a super large garbage bag to waterproof cushions. If you have a favorite chair or rug that you are afraid will be damaged, take the easy way out and put it where the person will not use it.

Sometimes people need help and are either unable to ask

for it or embarrassed to ask for it. People may have used children's words such as *pee, piss, tinkle,* or *take a leak,* or even obscure euphemisms such as *go for a walk.* The person with language problems may say "I want tea" or "take a peek." If the care giver (particularly someone unfamiliar with the patient) does not understand what the person is asking for, accidents can result. Learn what the person means and be sure that sitters or other care givers know also.

If the person is incontinent at night, limit the amount of fluid he drinks after supper unless there is some medical reason why he needs extra fluid. (The rest of the day, be sure he is getting plenty of fluids.) Get him up once at night. It may be helpful to get a bedside commode he can use easily, especially if he has trouble moving around. Night lights in the bathroom and bedroom greatly help, too.

Falls often occur on the way to the bathroom at night. Make sure there are adequate lights and no throw rugs, that the person can get out of bed, and that he has slippers that are not slippery or floppy.

A diary will provide you with the information you need to prevent many accidents. If you know when the person usually urinates (immediately upon awakening, about 10 A.M., an hour after he has his juice), you can take him to the toilet just before an accident would occur. This is, in fact, training yourself to the confused person's natural schedule. Many families find that they can tell when the patient needs to go to the bathroom. He may get restless or pick at his clothes. Routinely take him to the toilet every two to three hours. A regular schedule will avoid most "accidents," reduce skin irritations, and make life easier for you.

Certain nonverbal signals that tell us it is time or not time to urinate may influence some impaired people. Taking down one's underpants or opening one's fly, or sitting down on a toilet seat is a clue to "go." Dry clothes, and being in bed or in public are signals to "not go." (Some people are unable to urinate when there are "no go" clues, such as in the presence of another person or into a bedpan.) Taking down panties to undress a woman may cause her to urinate. You may be able to use such nonverbal clues to help a person go at the right time.

One man urinated every morning as soon as he put his feet on the floor. If this is what is happening, you may be able to be prepared and catch the urine in a urinal. There are urinals for women as well as men, but they may be hard to find. Use a plastic bowl for a standing woman. People may also be inhibited and unable to go when you are in the bathroom with them or if you ask them to use a commode in a room that is not a bathroom. It is often this involuntary "no go" response that leads families to say, "He wouldn't go when I took him and then he wet his pants. I think he is only being difficult."

Sometimes if a person has trouble urinating, it may help to give him a glass of water with a straw and ask him to blow bubbles. This seems to help the urine start.

Sometimes a person asks to go to the bathroom every few minutes. If this is a problem, it is helpful to have a urologist see the person to determine whether there is a medical reason why the person feels he needs to urinate frequently. A urinary tract infection or certain medications can give a person this feeling or can prevent his completely emptying his bladder. (If his bladder is not completely empty, he will soon feel the need to urinate again.) If you have ruled out medical reasons and are sure the person is emptying his bladder when he urinates, take him to the toilet every two to three hours and try to distract him in the interim period.

## Bowel Incontinence

Bowel incontinence, like urinary incontinence, should be discussed with the doctor. Temporary incontinence may be the result of an infection, diarrhea, or constipation. (See Chapter 6: "Medical Problems.")

Be sure that the bathroom is comfortable and that the person can sit without discomfort or instability long enough to move his bowels. His feet should rest on the floor and he should have something to hold onto. A bar, made from a broom handle and crossing in front of the person between two professionally installed supports, will give him something to hold and will encourage a restless person to stay put. Try giving him something to do or letting him listen to music.

Learn when the person usually moves his bowels and take him to the toilet at that time. Using a stool softener such as Metamucil will help.

Avoid reprimanding the person who has accidents.

## Cleaning Up

A person who remains in soiled or wet clothing can quickly develop skin irritations and sores. It is important to watch for these. Keeping the skin clean and dry is really the best protection against skin problems. The skin must be washed after each accident. Powder will keep the skin dry. Using a catheter as a continuing way to manage incontinence should be avoided if possible.

The personal care of an incontinent person can seem degrading for him and unpleasant or disgusting to you. Therefore, some families have made a deliberate effort to use the clean-up time as a time to express affection. This can help to make a necessary task less unpleasant.

There is wearing apparel available for incontinent people. The doctor or nurse will help you decide what is right for you. Disposable adult diapers and plastic outer pants are sold in drug stores and can be ordered through catalog stores. Some are more comfortable and stay on better if regular underpants are worn over them. Because of the negative feeling about the word *diaper*, these products are advertised as "adult briefs." Some are made so that one size fits all; for others, size is by hip or waist measurement. The type of filler used determines how much urine the brief will absorb. Products with a "gelling property," or super-absorbent polymers, usually hold much more than fiber-filled materials.

There are both disposable and washable garments. Some washable garments are not lined with soft materials, so the protective layer comes in contact with the skin and is uncomfortable.

Many families find disposable liners are better because they hold larger volumes of urine. Liners with "gel" hold more urine with less bulk than fiber-filled materials.

Several products consist of an outer, washable pant that holds a disposable pad. The idea is a soft, cool material in which the absorbent pad tends to draw urine away from the crotch so that the person's skin feels dry. It is helpful if the garment is designed so the pad can be changed without lowering the garment and so the garment can be lowered for toileting. The leg of the pant should fit snugly to prevent leakage, but should not bind.

Garments that don't fit or that are too saturated may leak. Don't expect the garment to hold more than one urination. Pads may say how much fluid they will hold. One full bladder may empty eight to ten ounces (one cup) of urine.

There are adult diaper services in large cities which save you the burden of washing these garments.

Disposable pads are made to protect bedding, and you can also buy rubberized flannel baby sheets. These are much less unpleasant than the older rubber sheet you may remember from your childhood.

Use a draw sheet in bed. This is a regular sheet folded in half lengthwise and tucked in across the bed. It holds a plastic pad in place between it. Should the patient have an accident, you have only the draw sheet and the pad to change. Absorbent bed pads used in combination with a draw sheet and rubber pad will help keep the bed dry. Look for pads with a polymer (gelling) effect and an embossed back to keep them from slipping. Follow the manufacturer's washing and drying instructions.

## PROBLEMS IN WALKING AND BALANCE; FALLING

As the person's illness progresses, he may become stiff or awkward, and have difficulty getting out of a chair or out of bed. He may develop a stooped or leaning posture or a shuffling walk. He will need close supervision when he is at risk of falling.

> A family member writes, "His steps are very slow now. As he walks, he often raises his feet high, for he has little sense of space. He clutchs door frames or chairs. Sometimes he just grasps at the air. His gaze is unfocused, like that of a blind man. He stops in front of mirrors, and he talks and laughs with the images there."

> Another wife says, "He sometimes falls down. He trips over his own feet or just crumples up. But when I try to lift him—and he is a big man—he yells and struggles against me."

Any of these symptoms *may* be caused by medications. Discuss with the doctor the onset of any change in walking, posture, stiffness, repetitive motions, or falling. He needs to be sure that there is not a treatable cause for them, such as medications, a delirium, or a small stroke. These same symptoms will occur when the dementing process has damaged the areas of the brain which control muscle movements. But do not assume this as the cause until the doctor has eliminated other causes.

Watch for the time the person can no longer safely negotiate stairs, or when he trips or has other difficulties walking. If a person is unsteady on his feet, have him take your arm, rather than your grasping his, if he will. Hold your arm close to your body. This maximizes your ability to keep your balance. Or you may steady him by walking behind him and holding his belt.

Put away scatter rugs, which may slide when the person steps on them. Install hand rails, especially in the bathroom. Pad the steps with rug samples. Staple or tack down rug edges. Round off shelf corners or pad them with foam rubber scraps. Be sure that chairs or other furniture that the person tends to lean on are sturdy; put unstable or antique furniture away. Simplify traffic patterns. Get things out of the way in areas where the person usually walks. Stair rails in many homes are inadequately anchored, and will come loose if a person leans on them heavily. Have someone knowledgeable about carpentry check this out for you.

Some people can learn to use canes or walkers. Others will not be able to learn this new skill. A Posey restraint can help a person sit up in a chair if he cannot do so unassisted. (See p. 139.)

It is important that when you help the person, you don't hurt yourself or throw yourself off balance. A physical therapist can show you ways to assist a person without strain. Avoid leaning forward or bending over when you lift. If you must bend to lift something, bend at the knees, not at the waist. Take your time; accidents happen when you rush yourself or the confused person. If you lift a person, lift from under his arms in the armpit. Avoid pulling him up out of bed by the arms. Avoid trying to put an awkward or heavy person in the back seat of a two-door car.

When a person falls,

1. remain calm.
2. check to see if he is visibly injured or in pain.
3. avoid precipitating a catastrophic reaction, and

4. watch the person for signs of pain, swelling, bruises, agitation, or increased distress, and call the doctor if these symptoms appear or if you think there is any chance that he hit his head or hurt himself. Instead of trying to get her husband up, one wife trained herself to sit down on the floor with him. (Obviously this took an effort to calm her own distress.) She would pat him and chat with him gently until he calmed down. When he was relaxed she was able to encourage him to get himself up one step at a time rather than having to lift him.

## Wheelchairs

If the time comes when the person needs a wheelchair, your doctor or a visiting nurse can give you guidance in selecting one and using it. Appendix 1 lists several books with information about maneuvering wheelchairs. Wheelchairs vary, so you will want to select the right one for your needs.

# 6

## MEDICAL PROBLEMS

PEOPLE WITH DEMENTING ILLNESSES can also suffer from other diseases ranging from relatively minor problems like the flu to serious illnesses. They may not be able to tell you they are in pain (even if they are able to speak well) or they may neglect their bodies. Cuts, bruises, or even broken bones can go unnoticed. People who sit or lie for long periods of time may develop pressure sores. Their physical health may gradually decline. *Correction of even minor physical problems can greatly help people who suffer dementing illnesses.*

You may have experienced a feeling of mental "dullness" when you are sick. This phenomenon can be worse in the demented person, whose system seems to be especially vulnerable to additional troubles. A delirium can be brought about by other conditions (flu, a minor cold, pneumonia, heart trouble, reactions to medications, and many other things) and it may look like a sudden worsening of the dementia. However, the delirium (and the symptoms) usually goes away when the

109

condition is treated. You should check routinely for signs of illness or injury and call them to the attention of your doctor.

All indications of pain or illness must be taken seriously. It is important to find a physician who is gentle, who understands the patient's condition, and who will take care of general medical problems. Do not let a doctor dismiss a patient because she is "senile" or "old." Insist that her infection be treated and her pains diagnosed and relieved. Because of the demented person's vulnerability to delirium, it is wise to check with the doctor about even minor conditions such as a cold.

Signals of illness include:

fever (temperature over 100° F.). When taking a temperature, be careful that the person does not bite the thermometer. You can use a paper thermometer that is placed on the forehead or you can get an approximate temperature by holding the thermometer in the person's armpit for three to five minutes.

flushing or paleness,

a rapid pulse over 100 (not obviously associated with exercise). Normal for most people is between 60 and 100 beats per minute. Have a nurse show you how to find a pulse in the wrist. Count for 20 seconds and multiply by 3. It is helpful to know what a normal pulse is for this individual.

vomiting or diarrhea,

changes in the skin (it may lose its elasticity, or look dry or pale),

dry, pale gums or sores in the mouth,

thirst or refusal of fluids or foods,

a change in personality, increased irritability, or increased lassitude or drowsiness.

headache,

an abrupt worsening of behavior, refusal to do certain

things she was previously willing to do. *(Behavior changes often signal illness.)*

moaning or shouting,

sudden onset of convulsions, hallucinations, or falls,

swelling of any part of the body (check especially hands and feet),

coughing, sneezing, signs of respiratory congestion, or difficulty breathing.

Ask yourself the following questions: Has the person had even a minor fall? Has she moved her bowels in the last seventy-two hours? Has she had a recent change in medication? Do mild pain killers such as aspirin relieve her? Does she have other health problems, such as heart disease, arthritis, or a cold?

If a person begins to lose weight, this may indicate the presence of a serious disease. It is important that your doctor determine the cause of any weight loss. A person who has lost 10 percent of her weight needs to be seen by a physician as soon as possible.

People who cannot express themselves well may not be able to answer yes or no when you ask them specific questions such as, "Does your head hurt?"

## PAIN

Families ask if people suffer pain as part of a dementing illness. As far as is known, Alzheimer's disease does not cause pain and multi-infarct dementia causes pain only very rarely. People with dementing illnesses do suffer pain from other causes, such as stomach and abdominal cramps; constipation; hidden sprains or broken bones; sitting too long in one position; flu; arthritis; pressure sores, bruises, or cuts; sores or rashes resulting from poor hygiene; sore teeth or gums; clothes or shoes that rub or are too tight; and open pins. Indications of pain include a sudden worsening of

**111**

behavior, moaning or shouting, refusal to do certain things, and increased restlessness. All signals of pain must be taken seriously. If the person cannot tell you where or whether she is in pain, a physician may have to search for a cause of the pain.

## FALLS AND INJURIES

People with dementing illnesses may become clumsy. They can fall out of bed, bump into things, trip, or cut themselves. It is easy to overlook serious injuries for several reasons: (1) older people are more vulnerable to broken bones from seemingly minor injuries, (2) they may continue to use a fractured limb, (3) demented people may not tell you they are in pain, or (4) even minor head injuries can cause bleeding within the skull, which must be treated promptly to avoid further brain damage.

Check the person routinely for cuts, bruises, and blisters that may be caused by accidents, falls, pacing, or uncomfortable clothing. Changes in behavior may be your only clue to an injury.

## PRESSURE SORES

Pressure sores (decubitus ulcers) develop when a person sits or lies down for prolonged periods, from tight clothing, swelling, or inadequate nutrition. Older people's skin may be quite sensitive to them. Pressure sores begin as red areas and can develop into open sores. They are more common over bony areas: heels, hips, shoulders, shoulder blades, spine, elbows, knees, buttocks, and ankles. You must watch for these, even in people who are able to walk, if the person spends a lot of time sitting or lying down. The doctor can show you how to treat existing sores. You will want to take steps to prevent further problems.

Encourage the person to change position: ask her to change the TV channel, go for a walk, set the table. Ask her to come into the kitchen to see if the cake is baking correctly or to come to the window to see something.

You can protect vulnerable areas if the person does not change position enough. Medical supply firms sell "floatation" cushions that the person can sit or lie on. (There are air cushions, water cushions, gel pads, foam pads, and combinations of these.) Select one that has soft, washable covers and shields against spills and odors. Stores also sell heel and elbow pads (these are made of a synthetic sheepskinlike material) that protect these bony areas.

## DEHYDRATION

Even people who can walk and appear to be able to care for themselves may become dehydrated. Because we assume that they are caring for themselves we may not watch for the signs of dehydration. Watch for this problem especially in people who have vomiting, diarrhea, or diabetes, or are taking diuretics (water pills) or heart medication. Symptoms include: thirst or refusal to drink; fever; flushing; rapid pulse; a dry, pale lining of the mouth or a dried, inelastic skin; dizziness or lightheadedness; and confusion or hallucinations.

The amount of fluid a person needs varies with the individual and with the season. People need more fluids during the summer months. If you are uncertain whether the person is getting enough fluid, ask your doctor how much the patient should be drinking.

## PNEUMONIA

Pneumonia is an infection of the lungs caused by a bacteria or virus. It is a frequent complication of dementia, but may be difficult to diagnose because symptoms such as fever or cough may be absent. Delirium may be the earliest symptom, so pneumonia should be suspected when a person with dementia worsens suddenly.

## CONSTIPATION

When a person is forgetful, she may not be able to remember when she last moved her bowels and she may not realize the cause of the discomfort that comes from constipation. Some people move their bowels less frequently than other people; however, they should have a bowel movement every two or three days.

Constipation can cause discomfort or pain, which can cause a worsening of the person's confusion. Constipation can lead to a bowel impaction, in which the bowel becomes partially or completely blocked and the body is unable to rid itself of wastes. You should consult a doctor or nurse if you suspect this. (A person can have diarrhea accompanying a partial impaction.)

Many factors contribute to the development of constipation. One important factor is that most Americans eat a diet high in refined, easy-to-prepare foods and low in fiber-containing foods that encourage bowel activity. Often when a person has a dementing illness or her dentures fit poorly or her teeth hurt, she makes further changes in her diet that aggravate the problem of constipation. The muscles of the bowel that move wastes along are believed to be less active as we age, and when we are less physically active, our bowel is even less active. Some drugs and some diet supplements (given to people who are not eating) tend to increase constipation.

If a person has a dementing illness, you cannot assume that she is able to keep track of when she last moved her bowels even if she seems to be only mildly impaired or if she tells you she is taking care of herself. If a confused person is living alone, she may have stopped eating things that take preparation skills and may be eating too much cake, cookies, and other low-fiber, highly refined foods. Since you do not live with her, it may be impossible to find out how regularly her bowels move. If you suspect that she may be getting constipated, you will need to keep track for her. Do this as quietly and unobtrusively as possible, so that you do not inadvertently make her feel that you are "taking over."

Most people are private about their bodily functions and a confused person can react angrily to your seeming invasion of her privacy. Also, keeping track of someone else's bowel movements is distasteful to many of us, and we tend to avoid doing it. These two feelings can conspire to cause a potentially serious problem to be overlooked.

When a demented person cannot talk and appears to be in pain or has a headache, do not overlook constipation as a possible cause. In the midst of providing care for a seriously impaired person, it is easy to forget to keep track of bowel movements. If you think the person may be constipated, you may want to talk this over with the doctor. He can quickly determine whether the person's bowels are working properly, and, if they are not, he can help manage the problem.

Regular or frequent use of laxatives is not recommended. Instead, increase the amount of fiber and water in the diet, and help the person get more exercise (perhaps a daily walk). The person should drink at least eight glasses of water or juice every day. Increase the amounts of vegetables (try putting them out as nibbles), fruits (including prunes, apples as more nibbles, or on cereal), whole-grain cereals (bran, whole-grain bread, whole-grain breakfast cereal), and salads, beans, and nuts she eats. Granola and other whole-grain cereals make a good snack.

Ask your doctor whether you should add more fiber by giving psyllium preparations (sold under various brand names, such as Metamucil). Do not use any such product without medical supervision.

## MEDICATIONS

Medications are a two-edged sword. They may play a vital part in helping the patient to sleep, in controlling her agitation, or in the treatment of other conditions. At the same time, people suffering from a dementing illness (and other people in general) are vulnerable to overmedication and to reactions from combinations of drugs. A sudden increase in agitation, a slow stooped walk, falling, drowsiness, incontinence, leaning, stiffness, or strange mouth or hand movements may be a side effect of medication and should be called to the doctor's attention. Physicians cannot always eliminate all the side effects of the medication and at the same time get the needed results. You and your physician must work together to achieve the best possible balance.

Your pharmacist is highly trained in the effects and interactions of drugs. Some pharmacists now have special training in geriatric pharmacology. Much of the responsibility for medications, however, will fall to you. Here are some ways you can help.

Be sure that all of the physicians involved in the person's care know about all of the medications she is taking. Sometimes combinations of drugs can make her confusion worse. You may want to take all the patient's prescription drugs and over-the-counter medications to your pharmacist and ask him to make up a card listing all of them. Ask the pharmacist if any of these medications should be listed on the patient's identification bracelet. (Also see the Medic Alert information in Appendix 3.)

Some drugs must be taken before meals, some after. Some have a cumulative effect (that is, they gradually build up their effectiveness) in the body, some don't. Older people and people with dementing illness are especially sensitive to incorrect dosages, so it is imperative that you see that the patient gets her medications in the amounts and at the times the doctor specifies.

Some patients do not understand why you want them to take a medication and may have a catastrophic reaction. Avoid arguing about it. Instead, tell the person one step at a time what is happening: "This is your pill. Dr. Brown gave it to you. . . . Put it in your mouth. . . . Drink some water. . . . Good." If the person becomes upset, try again later to give her her medicine. Some people will take pills more easily if you routinely put each dose in a cup or envelope instead of handing the person the whole bottle.

Patients may fail to swallow pills (or refuse). They may carry the pill around in their mouth and spit it out later. You may find the pills much later on the floor. Getting the person to drink something with the medication helps. If this continues to be a problem, ask the doctor if the medication is available in another form. Pills or a liquid may be easier to get down than capsules. Sometimes the pills can be crushed and mixed into food; applesauce works well. If you are not sure whether a person actually took her pill, find out from the doctor or the pharmacist what you should do. If pills are going on the floor, be sure that grandchildren or pets don't find and swallow them.

*Never* assume that a forgetful person is able to manage her own medications. If you must leave a person alone, put out one dose for her and take the bottle away with you. Even people with mild memory impairments (and sometimes normal people) forget whether they have taken their pills.

When you are tired or upset, you may forget the person's pills. Drug stores sell plastic containers with compartments labeled "Monday," "Tuesday," "Wednesday," etc. You can tell at a glance whether today's pills have been taken. (This device is helpful for *you*: do not trust the patient to be able to use it.) You can ask the pharmacist for easy-to-open pill bottles if the child-proof ones are difficult for you to open.

However, the child-proof caps may keep the confused person from taking pills she should not have.

Store medications where the confused person cannot reach them.

## DENTAL PROBLEMS

It is important that the person receive regular dental check-ups. Sores in her mouth may be hard for you to find and she may not be able to tell you about them. She may refuse to let you look in her mouth. Even mildly forgetful people may neglect their dentures and develop oral infections. The person's teeth must be pain-free or her dentures must fit well. Poor teeth or ill-fitting dentures can lead to poor nutrition, which can significantly add to her problems.

## VISION PROBLEMS

Sometimes it appears that the person cannot see well or is going blind. She may bump into things, pick her feet up very high over low curbs, be unable to pick up her food on her fork, or become confused or lost in dim light. One of several things may be happening. She may have a problem with her eyes such as farsightedness or cataracts. Have her checked by an ophthalmologist. A correctable vision problem should be corrected if possible so that her impaired brain can get the best possible information from her eyes. If she is both not seeing well and not thinking well, she will be even less able to make sense out of her environment and will function more poorly. Do not let a physician dismiss her vision problems because she is "senile." Even if he cannot help, he should explain to you what the problem is.

Brain-impaired people may be less able to distinguish between similar color intensities. Thus, light blue, light green, and light yellow may all look similar. A white handrail on a white wall may be hard to see. It may be hard for some people to tell where a light green wall joins a blue green carpet. This may cause the person to stumble into walls.

Some people have difficulty with depth perception. Prints and patterns may be confusing. A black and white bathroom floor can look as if it is full of holes. It may be difficult to know whether one is close enough to a chair to sit down. It may be hard to tell how high a step or curb is. It can be difficult to see where to step on stairs. Glare from a window tends to obliterate the detail of objects near it. The older eye may adjust more slowly to sudden changes from bright light to darkness or vice versa.

When the brain is not working well the person will be less able to compensate for these vision problems, but you can help her. She needs to see as well as possible so that she can function at her best level. Paint a handrail dark if the wall is light. Paint baseboards dark if the walls are light. The dark line will help the person see the change from floor to wall. Cover the bathroom with washable carpeting that is secured so that it does not slip. Delineate the edges and bottom of the bathtub with colorful strips of waterproof tape. Paint stair risers and treads contrasting colors. The contrast will help. Outline doors, mantelpieces, and other things the person bumps into with bright tape in a contrasting color and color intensity (light on dark or dark on light).

Increase the light in rooms in the daytime and evening and leave nightlights on at night. Install lights in dark closets. Cover chairs in bright, contrasting colors without patterns. Put a towel or spread over the chair if you don't want to recover it. Leave chairs in their familiar places.

People with dementing illnesses can also lose the ability to *know* what they see. In this instance the eyes work all right but the brain is no longer correctly using what the eyes tell it. For example, the person may bump into furniture, not because she has a vision problem but because her brain is not working properly. What seem like vision problems may be part of the dementia. This condition is called agnosia and is discussed in Chapter 8. When problems are caused by agnosia, the ophthalmologist will not be able to help. In fact, it may be difficult for him to test the vision of a person with thinking or language impairments. Obviously, when this is the problem, it will do no good to tell the person to watch where she is going. She will need increasing care to protect her from injuries she cannot avoid, and you may need to check her frequently for cuts and bruises.

If the person is laying her glasses down and forgetting them, it often helps to have her wear them on a chain. Keep her old glasses, or buy her a spare pair in case she loses her glasses. Carry her prescription and your own with you if you go out of town. With a prescription, you can replace lost or broken glasses with less trouble and expense.

If the person wears contact lenses, you may need to replace them with glasses before the person reaches a point where she is unable to manage contact lenses. If she continues to wear lenses, you must watch for irritations to the eye and be sure she cares for her lenses properly.

## HEARING PROBLEMS

Failing to hear properly deprives the confused brain of information needed to make sense of the environment, and hearing loss can cause or worsen suspiciousness or withdrawal (see Chapter 8). It is important to correct any hearing loss if possible. A physician can determine the cause of the hearing loss and help you select an appropriate hearing aid. As with vision problems, it can be difficult for you to separate problems in thinking from problems in hearing. Since the ill person cannot learn easily, she may not be able to adjust to her hearing aid. (Hearing aids pick up background noises, which can sound loud and be upsetting to the wearer.) You may want to purchase a hearing aid with the agreement that you can return it if it does not work out.

If the person uses a hearing aid, you must be responsible for it and must check regularly to see that the batteries are working.

In addition to correcting the loss with a hearing aid, here are some things you can do:

1. Reduce background noises, such as noise from appliances, the television, or several people talking at once. It is difficult for the impaired person to distinguish between these and what she wants to hear.

2. Lower the pitch of your voice. High-frequency sounds are harder to hear.

3. Give the person clues to where sounds are coming from. It can be hard to locate and identify sounds, and this may confuse the person. Remind her, "That is the sound of the garbage truck."

4. Use several kinds of clues at one time: point, speak, and gently guide the person, for example.

## VISITING THE DOCTOR

Visits to the doctor or dentist can turn into an ordeal for you and the patient. Here are some ways to make them easier.

The forgetful person may not be able to understand where she is going or why. This, combined with the bustle of getting ready to go, may precipitate a catastrophic reaction. Look for ways to simplify things for her.

Some people do better if they know in advance that they are going to the doctor. Others do better if you avoid an argument by not bringing up the doctor visit until you are almost there. Instead of saying, "We have to get up early today. Hurry with your breakfast because today is your visit to Dr. Brown, and he has to change your medicine," just get the person up with no comment, serve her breakfast, and help her into her coat. When you are almost there, say, "We are seeing Dr. Brown today."

Rather than get in an argument, ignore or downplay objections.

121

If the person says, "I am not going to the doctor," instead of saying, "You have to go to the doctor," try changing the subject and saying something like "We will get an ice cream while we are downtown."

Plan your trip in advance. Know where you are going, where you will park, how long it will take, and whether there are stairs or elevators. Allow enough time without rushing, but not so much time that you will be early and have a longer wait. Ask for an appointment at the person's best time of day. Take someone with you to help while you drive.

Talk to the receptionist or nurse. She may be able to tell you whether you have a long wait. If the office is crowded and noisy, she may be able to arrange for you to wait in a quieter place. Take along some snacks, a package of instant soup (the receptionist can get you hot water), or some activity the person enjoys doing. If the receptionist knows that you have a long wait, you may be able to take a short walk if you check in frequently with her. Never leave a forgetful person alone in the waiting room. The strange place may upset her or she may wander away.

The doctor may prescribe a sedative for the patient if other methods fail. Usually, however, your being calm and matter of fact and giving the person simple information and reassurance are all that is needed.

## SEIZURES, FITS, OR CONVULSIONS

The majority of people with dementing illnesses do not develop seizures. Because they are so uncommon, you are not likely to have to face this problem. However, seizures can be frightening for you if you are not prepared to deal with them. Various diseases can cause seizures. Therefore, if the person does have a seizure it may not be related to the dementia.

There are several types of seizure. In a generalized tonic-clonic seizure (the kind we usually associate with a fit or seizure), the person becomes rigid, falls, and loses consciousness. Her breathing can become irregular or even stop briefly. Then her muscles will begin to jerk and she may clench her teeth tightly. After some seconds the jerking will stop and the person will slowly regain consciousness. She may be confused, sleepy, or have a headache. She may have difficulty talking.

Other types of seizure are less dramatic. For example, just a hand or arm may move in a repetitive manner.

A single seizure is not life-threatening. Most important, remain calm. Do not try to restrain the person. Try to protect her from falling or banging her head on something hard. If she is on the floor, move things out of the way. If she is seated you may be able to ease her to the floor or quickly push a sofa cushion under her to soften her fall if she should fall out of the chair.

Do not try to move her or stop the seizure. Stay with her and let the seizure run its course. Do not try to hold the tongue and do not try to put a spoon in the patient's mouth. Never force her mouth open after her teeth are clenched. You may damage her teeth and gums. Loosen clothing if you can. For example, unfasten a belt, a necktie, or buttons at the neckline.

When the jerking has ceased, be sure the person is breathing correctly. If she has more saliva than usual, turn her head gently to the side and wipe out her mouth. Let her sleep or rest if she wishes. She may be confused or irritable or even combative after the seizure. She may know something is wrong, but she will not remember the seizure. Be calm, gentle, and reassuring. Avoid restraining her, restricting her, or insisting on what she should do.

Take a few minutes after the seizure to relax and collect yourself.

If the person has a partial seizure nothing need be done. If the person wanders about, follow her and try to prevent her from hurting herself. When this type of seizure ends she may be temporarily confused, irritable, or have trouble talking. You may be able to identify the warning signals that a seizure is starting, such as specific repetitive movements. If so, you can make sure the person is in a safe place (out of traffic, away from stairs or stoves, etc.).

Your doctor can be helpful with seizures. He should be called the first time the person has any type of seizure, so that he can check her and determine the cause of the seizure. Stay with the person until the seizure is over and you have had a chance to collect yourself. Then call the doctor. He can prescribe medication to minimize the likelihood of further seizures.

If the patient is being treated for seizures, the doctor should be called if the person has many seizures over a short period of time, if the symptoms do not go away after several hours, or if you suspect that the person has hit her head or injured herself in some other way.

Seizures are frightening and unpleasant to watch, but they are usually not life-threatening nor are they indications of danger to others or of insanity. They can become less frightening for you as you learn how to respond to them. Find a nurse or experienced family member with whom you can discuss your distress and who can knowledgeably reassure you.

## JERKING MOVEMENTS (MYOCLONUS)

Patients with Alzheimer's disease occasionally develop rapid jerking movements of their arms, legs, or body. These are called myoclonic jerks. They are not seizures; seizures are repeated movements of the same muscles, while myoclonic jerks are single thrusts of an arm or of the head.

Myoclonic jerks are not a cause for alarm. They do not progress to seizures. The only danger they may cause would be inadvertent hitting of something and possible accidental injury. At present there are no good treatments for the myoclonus associated with Alzheimer's disease. Drugs can be tried but these usually have significant side effects and offer little improvement.

## THE DEATH OF THE IMPAIRED PERSON

Whenever you have the responsibility for an ill or elderly person, you face the possibility of that person's death. You may have questions you are reluctant to bring up with the doctor. Often thinking about such things in advance will help relieve your mind and can make things easier if you have to face a crisis.

### Cause of Death

In the final stages of a progressive dementing illness, so much of the nervous system is failing that this profoundly effects the rest of the body. The person may be confined to bed, incontinent, and aphasic. The *immediate* cause of death is often a complicating condition such as pneumonia, malnutrition (these people sometimes stop eating), dehydration, or infection. Death certificates often list only this immediate cause of death and do not list the dementing illness as a cause of death. This has made it difficult for epidemiologists to determine accurately how prevalent dementing illnesses are.

### Dying at Home

Families sometimes worry that the ill or elderly person will die at home, perhaps in her sleep, and that they will find her. Because of this a care giver may be afraid to sleep soundly or may get up to check on the sick person several times a night.

*One daughter said, "I don't know what I would do. What if one of the children found her?"*

Perhaps you have heard of someone who found a husband or wife dead, and you wonder how you would handle this. Most families find it reassuring to know what to do. Select a funeral director or mortician in advance. Should a death occur, you have only to call him or your doctor.

In some areas there are special resources for people who have terminal illnesses and who, with their families, wish to die at home or in a hospice. Your hospital will know about hospices and other programs in your area. Hospice programs may be able to give you information about how to plan for a death and some advice and counseling.

## Prolonging Suffering?

There is another aspect to consider when a person has a slow, chronic, terminal illness: the question of whether it would be better to allow life to end rather than prolong suffering. This is a serious question, one doctors, judges, and ministers struggle with as well as the seriously ill and their families. Each of us must make that decision for himself based on his unique background, beliefs, and experiences.

Talking about death is often difficult. Yet, getting these thoughts out in the open by talking with other family members, friends, a minister, or a doctor can often relieve us of the oppressive thought that we are alone. Such thoughts of death often reflect our underlying feelings of depression, anger, or hopelessness, and talking about our concerns can be a bridge to these emotions.

## Autopsy

Your doctor may ask you for permission to perform an autopsy or you may decide to request one. We feel that it is important for autopsies to be performed for several reasons. First, an autopsy is the only way to confirm a diagnosis of Alzheimer's disease and many other causes of dementia. It can be reassuring to you to know the exact illness. In the future such knowledge may be important when specific therapies are available. Also, individual physicians frequently learn from the autopsies information that they can use to help others. Finally, autopsy studies advance our knowledge of the dementing illnesses. If you are near an institution that is conducting research in dementia, an autopsy may be helpful to the scientists there. Autopsies do not disfigure the body.

You can obtain information about how and where to arrange for an autopsy from the Alzheimer's Disease and Related Disorders Association.

# 7

## PROBLEMS OF BEHAVIOR

### CONCEALED MEMORY LOSS

PEOPLE WITH A DETERIORATING DEMENTING DISEASE can become skillful at hiding their declining abilities and forgetfulness. This is understandable; no one wants to admit that he is getting "senile."

This tendency to hide limitations can be distressing for families. The person living with someone suffering from a dementing illness may know that the person is impaired yet get no support or understanding from others who cannot see the problem. Friends may say that "he looks and sounds perfectly all right. I don't see anything wrong, and I don't see why he cannot remember to call me." Family members may not be able to differentiate between real memory loss and plain contrariness.

When a person has been living alone, family, neighbors, and friends may be unaware for a long time that anything is wrong. When the person denies that he has any memory problems, he may manage for years until a crisis occurs. Families are often shocked and distressed by the extent of the problem when they finally learn of it.

You may wonder what the person is still able to do for himself and what needs to be done for him. If he is still employed, has responsibility for his own money, or is driving, he may not realize or may be unwilling to admit that he can no longer manage these tasks as well as he once could. Some people recognize that their memory is slipping. Different people cope with this in different ways. While some people don't want to admit that anything is wrong, others find relief and comfort in talking about what is happening to them. Listen to their thoughts, feelings, and fears if this is so. This can be comforting and can give you a chance to correct misconceptions.

Others may successfully conceal their impairment by keeping lists. They may use conversational devices, such as saying "Of course I know that" to cover their forgetfulness. Some people get angry and blame others when they forget things. Some people stop participating in activities that they have always enjoyed.

A frequent characteristic of the dementing illnesses is that personality and social skills appear nearly intact while memory and the ability to learn are being lost. This condition enables a person to conceal his illness for a long time. One can talk with such a person about routine matters and fail to recognize that his memory or thinking is impaired. Psychological testing or an occupational therapy evaluation can be helpful in such situations because the evaluation will give you a realistic measure of how much you can expect from the impaired individual and what things the person can still do. Because dementing illnesses can be so deceiving, even to people close to the person, the assessment these professionals can give is most important to you in helping you and your family plan realistically. These professionals may also talk over their findings with the impaired person and show him ways he can remain as independent as possible.

## WANDERING

Wandering is a common and frequently serious problem that deserves thoughtful consideration. Wandering behavior can make it difficult to manage a person at home. It can make it impossible for day care centers or nursing homes to care for a person. The impaired person is endangered when he wanders into busy streets or into strange neighborhoods. When a confused person becomes disoriented and lost, he may feel frightened. Because so many people do not understand dementia, strangers who try to help may think the individual is drunk or insane. When wandering occurs at night it can deprive the family of needed rest. However, often it can be stopped or at least reduced.

Since it appears that there are different kinds of wandering and different reasons why brain-impaired people wander, identifying the cause of the behavior may help you plan a strategy to manage it.

Wandering may result from getting lost. Sometimes a person sets out on an errand, such as going to the store, makes a wrong turn, becomes disoriented, and gets completely lost trying to find his way back. Or he may go shopping with you, lose sight of you, and get lost trying to find you.

Wandering often increases when a person moves to a new home, begins a day care program, or for some other reason is in a new environment.

Some people wander around intermittently for no apparent reason.

Some wandering behavior appears aimless and can go on for hours. It appears different from the wandering associated with being lost or with being in a new place. Some people develop an agitated, determined pacing. When this continues it gets on everyone's nerves. It can be dangerous when the person is determined to get away. This seemingly incomprehensible pacing may be associated with the damage to the brain. Occasionally, continuous pacing and wandering can cause the person's feet to swell.

Some people wander at night. This can be dangerous for the impaired person and exhausting for you. Night wandering can have different causes, from simple disorientation to agitated pacing.

Many of us can sympathize with the confused person's experience of becoming disoriented. We may have lost our car at a parking lot or gotten "turned around" in a strange place. For a few minutes we feel unnerved until we get hold of ourselves and work out a logical way to find out where we are. The person with a memory impairment is more likely to panic, is less able to "get hold of himself," and may feel that he must keep his disorientation a secret.

When wandering is made worse by a move to a new home or by some other change in the environment, it may be because it is difficult for a confused, memory-impaired person to learn his way around in a new setting. He may not be able to understand that he has moved and is determined to go "home." The stress of such a change may impair his remaining abilities, which makes it harder for him to learn his way around.

Aimless wandering may be the person's way of saying, "I *feel* lost. I am searching for the things I feel I have lost." Sometimes wandering behavior is the person's way of trying to communicate feeling.

*Mr. Griffith was a vigorous man of sixty who kept leaving the day care center. The police would pick him up several miles away hiking down the highway. Mr. Griffith always explained that he was going to Florida. Florida represented home, friends, security, and family to Mr. Griffith.*

Wandering may be the person's way of expressing restlessness, boredom, or the need for exercise. It may help to fill the need of an active person to be "doing something."

A constant or agitated pacing or a determination to get away may be difficult to manage. Sometimes this is a catastrophic reaction. Something may be upsetting the person. He may not be able to make sense out of his surroundings or may be misinterpreting what he sees or hears. Sometimes this agitated wandering appears to be a direct result of the brain damage. It is hard to know exactly what is happening to the brain, but we do know that brain function can be seriously and extensively disrupted. Remind yourself that this is not a behavior that the person can control.

Night wandering can also have various causes, from simple disorientation to a seemingly incomprehensible part of the brain injury (see p. 140).

## Management of Wandering

The management of wandering behavior depends on the cause of the wandering. If the person is getting lost and if you are sure he can still read and follow instructions, a pocket card may help him. Write *simple* instructions on a card he can carry in his pocket and refer to if he is lost. You might put at the top of the card the written reminder "stay calm and don't walk away." You might write on the card "call home" and put the telephone number, or write "ask a clerk to show you to the men's wear department and stay there. I will come for you." You may need different cards for different trips. This will make it possible for a mildly confused person to help himself.

It is essential that you get the person a necklace or bracelet with his name and your phone number on it, and the statement "memory impaired." A bracelet that is securely fastened (so the patient cannot take it off) and too small to slip off is probably safer than a necklace. This information will help anyone who finds the person if he gets lost. You can have an inexpensive bracelet engraved in a store that engraves mugs, key rings, etc. Have a "memory impaired" bracelet made *now* if there is any possibility that the person will wander or get lost. This is so important that some clinics require that their patients have such identification. A lost, confused person will be afraid and upset, and this can cause him to resist help. He may be ignored or assumed to be crazy by the people around him. Under stress he may function more poorly than he usually does.

There are also Medic Alert bracelets. (See Appendix 3 for ordering information.) You may want the person to wear one of these, especially if he has a heart condition or some other serious health problem. The Medic Alert bracelet gives a toll-free number that a hospital can call for medical information on the person. This is slower than reading a custom-made bracelet, and the bracelet may not be checked by the person trying to help.

Some forgetful people will carry a card in their pocket or wallet which gives their name, address, and phone number. Others will lose it or throw it away. However, ID cards are worth trying.

To reduce increased wandering when the person moves to a new environment, you may want to plan in advance of the move to make it as easy as possible for the impaired person. When a person is still able to understand and participate in what is going on around him, it may help to introduce him gradually to his new situation. If he is moving to a new home, involve him in planning the move (see p. 66) and visit often in the new setting before he moves. When a person's impairment makes it impossible for him to understand what is happening, it may be easier not to introduce him gradually but simply to make the move as quietly and with as little fuss as possible. Each person is unique. Try to balance his need to participate in decision making with his ability to understand.

If the person is going to attend a day care center, you might go with him the first time, or have him spend only a few hours rather than a full day there the first few times. This will help him realize that you want him to be in the center.

When a confused person finds himself in a new place, he may feel that he is lost, that you cannot find him, or that he is not supposed to be where he is. Reassure the disoriented person often about where he is and why he is there. "You have come to live with me, Father. Here is your room with your things in it," or "You are at the day care center. You will go home at 3:00."

Families tell us "It doesn't work!" when we give this advice. It doesn't work in the sense that the person may continue to insist that he doesn't live here and keep trying to wander away. This is because he is memory impaired and does not remember what you told him. He still needs to be gently and frequently reassured about his whereabouts. It takes time and patience to get him to accept the move and gradually come to feel secure. He also needs this frequent reassurance that you know where he is. A gentle reassurance and your understanding of his confusion help reduce his fear and the number of catastrophic reactions he has. Our experience with people who are hospitalized for their dementia is that, even with difficult people, frequent gentle reassurance about where they are sometimes helps them become comfortable (and easier to manage). However, this may take several (five to seven) days.

A move often upsets a person with a dementing illness, causing him to wander more or making his behavior worse for a period of time. It is helpful to know that this is usually a temporary crisis.

Because changes may make the person's behavior or wandering worse, it is important to consider changes carefully. You may decide that a vacation or an extended visit is not worth upsetting the confused person.

When the wandering seems to be aimless, some professionals suspect that exercise helps to reduce this restlessness. Try taking the person for a long, vigorous walk each day. You may have to continue an activity plan for several weeks before you see whether it is making a difference.

When wandering seems to be the person's way of saying, "I *feel* lost" or "I am searching for the things I feel I have lost," you can help by surrounding the person with familiar things, for example, pictures of his family. Make him feel welcome by talking with him or by taking time to have a cup of tea with him.

An agitated pacing or determined efforts to wander away are sometimes caused by frequent or almost constant catastrophic reactions. Ask yourself what may be happening that is precipitating catastrophic reactions. Does this behavior happen at about the same time each day? Does it happen each time the person is asked to do a certain thing (like take a bath)? Review the way people around the confused person are responding to his wandering. Does their response increase his restlessness and wandering? If you must restrain a person or go after him, try to distract him rather than directly confronting him. Talking calmly can reassure him and prevent a catastrophic reaction that will change aimless wandering into a determination to get away. Wandering can often be reduced by creating an environment that calms the person.

*When Mrs. Dollinger came into the hospital, she had been making constant, determined efforts to leave the nursing home. In the hospital, which was also a strange place, the nurses had much less difficulty with her.*

*In both places Mrs. Dollinger felt lost. She knew this*

*was not where she lived and she wanted to go home. Also, she was lonely; she wanted to go back to her job, where her fogged mind remembered friends and a sense of belonging. So she wandered toward the door. The overworked nursing staff at the nursing home would yell loudly to her "Come back here." After a few days, one of the other residents in the home began to "help." "Mrs. Dollinger escaped again!" she would shout. The noise confused Mrs. Dollinger, who doubled her efforts to get out. This brought a nurse on the run; Mrs. Dollinger would panic and run away as fast as she could, straight onto a busy street. When an attendant caught her arm and held her, Mrs. Dollinger bit him. This happened several times, exhausting the staff and precipitating almost constant catastrophic reactions. The family was told that Mrs. Dollinger was unmanageable.*

*In the hospital Mrs. Dollinger headed for the door almost at once. A nurse approached her quietly and suggested they have a cup of tea together (distraction rather than confrontation). Mrs. Dollinger never stopped wandering to the door, but her vigorous effort to escape and assaultive behavior did stop.*

Medication may reduce the patient's restlessness. However, some drugs can induce restlessness as a side effect. Medications must be closely supervised by a physician. Occasionally, the judicious use of major tranquilizers, under close medical supervision, can lessen wandering significantly.

If incessant wandering causes the person's feet to swell, try sitting down with him and helping him to put his feet up. He may sit still as long as you sit with him. Other measures (see p. 140) may be necessary if you cannot get him off his feet. Be sure to check with the doctor about swelling or injured feet. The discomfort can make the person's behavior worse.

Changing the environment to protect the person is an important part of coping with wandering. One family found that the confused person would not go outside if he did not have his shoes on. Taking his shoes away and giving him slippers kept him inside.

It is often helpful to install locks that are difficult to operate or that are unfamiliar to the confused person, so that he cannot go outside unsupervised. Sometimes inexpensive devices such as a spring-operated latch are sufficient because the impaired person cannot learn the new task of opening them. A confused person is less likely to look for a lock at the bottom of the door. Make sure you can operate the locks quickly in case of a fire. There is an inexpensive plastic gadget available in hardware stores called a child-proof knob. It slips over the existing door knob. You can still open the door, but the confused person cannot figure out how to operate it.

Check other means of exit as well as doors. Confused people may climb out second story windows. Secure locks protect you as well as ensure the person's safety. The police department can advise you about inexpensive ways to secure your windows and patio doors.

If the person does go outside, be alert to hazards in the neighborhood such as busy streets, swimming pools, or dogs. The person may no longer possess the *judgment* to protect himself from these things. You may want to take a walk through the neighborhood in which the person lives and look around thoughtfully for things that are dangerous for a person who no longer has the ability to assess his surroundings appropriately. At the same time you may want to alert people in the neighborhood to the problem, reassuring them that the person is not crazy or dangerous but just disoriented.

The person himself can be his own worst hazard. When he looks healthy and acts reasonable, people tend to forget that he may have lost the judgment that would keep him from stepping over the side of a swimming pool or in front of a car.

Other people are also an environmental hazard to the confused person who wanders. In addition to those who don't understand are the cruel and vicious who seek out the elderly and the frail in order to harass, torment, or rob them. Unfortunately, there seem to be enough such people, even in the "nicest" neighborhoods, for you to recognize this hazard and protect the confused person from them.

There are physical devices to restrain a person in a chair or bed. The decision to use a restraint should be made jointly between you and the health care professional who knows the person best, and these *should be used only after all other possibilities have been tried*. (We are addressing here the use of restraints at home. The use of restraints in a nursing home involves other issues and will be discussed in Chapter 16.) The most familiar restraint is the Posey restraint. A patient can turn, shift position, or roll to the side in a Posey. Poseys can be rented from a medical supply house. It is very important that it be properly applied; a nurse should show you how to use it.

A gerichair is like a recliner with a tray on it that prevents the person from getting up. It will elevate a person's feet. A person can eat, do crafts, or watch television in gerichair. These can also be rented or purchased.

Nurses occasionally find that a restraint, especially at night, provides the person with a firm reassurance that he must stay where he is. However, restraints further agitate some people.

Either a chair or a Posey restraint may help to keep a person still and safe long enough for you to take a bath or fix supper. Using restraints or a chair gives the person's feet a chance to recover.

Very agitated people can hurt themselves fighting against the bed while in restraints or may tip over a chair in which they are restrained. People cannot be left unsupervised for long periods in either Poseys or gerichairs. *Never* leave a person alone in the house while he is restrained, because of the possibility of a fire.

People with dementing illnesses can be difficult to manage and wandering can be a serious problem. The responses vary with each person. One confused lady was only looking for the bathroom when she wandered away. A sign solved the problem. Another man got a screwdriver and took the door off its hinges when he found that he could not operate the lock.

You may reach a point when the wandering behavior is more than you can manage or when a person cannot be kept safely in a home setting. If this time comes, you will have done all you can, and will need to plan realistically for institutional care for the person. Many places will not accept a patient who is agitated, combative, or a wanderer. See Chapter 16 for a discussion of placement issues.

## SLEEP DISTURBANCES; NIGHT WANDERING

Many people with dementing illnesses are restless at night. They may wake to go to the bathroom and become confused and disoriented in the dark. They may wander around the house, get dressed, try to cook, or even go outside. They may ''see things'' or ''hear things'' that are not there. Few things are more distressing than having your much-needed sleep disrupted night after night. Fortunately, there are ways to reduce this behavior.

Older people seem to need less sleep than younger people. People with dementing illnesses may not be getting enough exercise to make them tired at night, or they may be dozing during the day. Often it seems that the internal ''clock'' within the brain is damaged by the dementing illness. Some nighttime behavior problems may be in response to dreams that the impaired person cannot separate from reality.

If the person is napping during the day he will be less tired at night. Try to keep him occupied, active, and awake in the daytime. If he is getting tranquilizing drugs to control his behavior, these may be making him drowsy during the day. Discuss with the doctor the possibility of giving most of the tranquilizer in the evening instead of spreading the dose throughout the day. This may provide the behavior control without making the person sleepy during the day. If he must sleep during the day, try to get some rest yourself at the same time.

Often people with dementing illnesses are not very active and don't get much exercise. It may be helpful to plan a regular activity program—a long walk, for example—in the late afternoon. This may make the person tired enough to sleep better at night. A car ride makes some people sleepy.

See that the person has used the bathroom before going to sleep.

Older people may not see as well in the dark and this may add to their confusion. As our eyes age, it becomes more difficult to distinguish dim shapes in poor light. The confused person may misinterpret what he sees, so he thinks he sees people or thinks he is in some other place. This can cause catastrophic reactions. Leave a nightlight on in the bedroom and bathroom. Nightlights in other rooms may also help the person orient himself at night. Reflector tape around the bathroom door may help. Try renting a commode that can sit right beside the bed.

Many of us have had the experience of waking from a sound sleep and momentarily not knowing where we are. This may be magnified for the confused person. Your quiet reassurance may be all that is needed.

Be sure the sleeping arrangements are comfortable: the room is neither too warm nor too cool, and the bedding is comfortable. Quilts are less likely to tangle than blankets and sheets. Bedrails help some people remember they are in bed. Other people get upset and try to climb over them, which is dangerous. You may want to rent bedrails and see if they help. Bedrails are available for most beds.

If the confused person gets up in the night, speak softly and quietly to him. When you are awakened suddenly in the night, you may respond irritably and speak crossly. This may precipitate a catastrophic reaction in the impaired person, which will get everybody up in the middle of the night. Often all that is needed is gently to remind the person that it is still nighttime and that he should go back to bed. A person will often go back to sleep after he has had a cup of warm milk. Encourage him to go back to bed and sit with him quietly while he drinks his milk. A radio playing softly will quiet some people. Try using night-darkening shades and quietly remind the disoriented person that it is dark and the shades are drawn, therefore it is time to stay in bed.

Sometimes a person who will not sleep in bed will sleep in a lounge chair or on a sofa. If the person gets up in the night and gets dressed, he may sit back down again and fall asleep in his clothes if you don't interfere. It may be better to accept this than to be up part of the night arguing about it.

If the person does wander at night, you must examine your house for safety hazards. Arrange the bedroom so the person can move around safely. Lock the window. Can he turn on the stove or start a fire while you are sleeping? Can he unlock and walk out the outside doors? Can he, while trying to go to the bathroom, fall down the stairs? A gate across the stairs may be essential in houses where a disoriented person sleeps.

Finally, if these measures fail, sedative-hypnotics are helpful. However, you cannot simply give the person a sleeping pill and solve the problem. Sedatives affect the chemistry of the brain, which is complex and sensitive. Your doctor faces a series of difficult, interacting problems when he begins to prescribe sedatives.

Older people, including the well elderly, are more subject to side effects from drugs than are younger people. Side effects of sedatives are numerous and some are serious. Brain-injured people are more sensitive to drugs than well people. Older people are more likely to be taking other drugs that can interact with a sedative or to have other illnesses that can be aggravated by a sedative.

Sedating the person may make him sleep in the daytime instead of at night or it may have a hangover effect that worsens his cognitive functioning during the day. It can make him more confused, more vulnerable to falls, or incontinent. Paradoxically, it may even worsen sleep. Each person is different; what works for one may not work for another.

The effect of the sedative may change—for many reasons—after it has been used for a while. Your doctor may have to try first one drug and then another, carefully adjusting the dosage and the time at which it is given. Drugs may not make the person sleep all night. Therefore, it is important that you do all you can to help the person sleep with other methods. This does not mean that we discourage the use of sedatives; they are a very useful tool, but only one of several tools used to manage a difficult problem.

## WORSENING IN THE EVENING

People with dementing illnesses often seem to have more behavior problems in the evening. We do not know what causes this. It may be that the person cannot see clearly in dim light and misinterprets what he sees, causing catastrophic reactions. Leaving lights on often helps. Telling the person where he is and what is happening may help.

A whole day of trying to cope with confusing perceptions of the environment may be tiring, so a person's tolerance for stress is lower at the end of the day. You are also more tired and may subtly communicate your fatigue to the confused person, causing catastrophic reactions.

Plan the person's day so that fewer things are expected of

him in the evening. A bath (which is often difficult), for example, might be scheduled for morning or midafternoon if this works better.

Sometimes there are more things going on at once in the house in the evening. This may overstimulate the already confused and tired person. For example, are you turning on the TV? Are more people in the house in the evening? Are you busy fixing supper? Are children coming in? Being tired may make it harder for him to understand what is going on and may cause him to have catastrophic reactions.

If possible, try to reduce the number of things going on around the person at his worst times of day or try to confine the family activity to an area away from the impaired person. It is also important to try to plan your day so that you are reasonably rested and not too pressed for time at the times of day that you observe are worst for the confused person. For example, if he gets most upset while you are getting supper, try to plan meals that are quick and easy, that are left over from lunch, or that you can prepare in advance. Eat the larger meal at midday.

Sometimes the trouble is that the person wants your constant attention and becomes more demanding when you are busy with other things. Perhaps you can occupy the person with a simple chore close to you while you work, or get someone else in the family to spend some time with him.

You may want to talk to the doctor about changing the schedule for giving medications if other methods don't help change this pattern.

Periods of restlessness or sleeplessness may be an unavoidable part of the brain injury. Reassure yourself that the person is not doing this deliberately, even though it may seem like he acts up at the times of day that are hardest for you.

## LOSING THINGS AND HIDING THINGS

Most people with dementing illnesses put things down and forget where they put them. Others hide things and forget where they hid them. Either way, the result is the same; just when you need them most the person's dentures or your car keys have vanished and cannot be found.

First, remember that you probably cannot ask the impaired person where he put them. He will not remember, and you may precipitate a catastrophic reaction by asking him.

There are several things you can do to reduce this problem. A neat house makes it easier to locate misplaced items. It is almost impossible to find something hidden in a cluttered closet or drawer. Limit the number of hiding places by locking some closets or rooms.

Take away valuable items such as rings or silver so they cannot be hidden and lost. Do not keep a significant amount of cash around the house. Make small, easily lost items larger and/or more visible—for example, put a large attachment on your key ring. Have a spare set of necessary items such as keys, eyeglasses, and hearing aid batteries if at all possible.

Get in the habit of checking the contents of wastebaskets before you empty them. Check under mattresses, under sofa cushions, in wastebaskets, in shoes, and in everyone's bureau drawers for lost items. Ask yourself where the confused person used to put things for security. Where did he hide Christmas gifts or money? These are good places to look for lost dentures.

## INAPPROPRIATE SEXUAL BEHAVIOR

Sometimes confused people take off their clothes or wander out into the livingroom or down the street undressed. For example,

*One teenage boy came home to find his father sitting on the
back porch reading the newspaper. He was naked except
for his hat.*

Occasionally confused people will expose themselves in
public. Sometimes very confused people will fondle their
genitals. Or they will fidget in such a way that their fidgeting
reminds others of sexual behaviors, which is upsetting.

*One man repeatedly undid his belt buckle and unzipped his
trousers.*

*A woman kept fidgeting with the buttons of her blouse.*

Sometimes brain damage will cause a person to demand
sexual activities frequently or inappropriately. But much more
common than actual inappropriate sexual behavior is the myth
that "senile" people will develop inappropriate sexual behaviors.

*One wife who brought her husband to the hospital for care
confessed that she had no problems managing him but that
she had been told that, as he got worse, he would go into
his "second childhood" and start exposing himself to little
girls.*

There is *no* basis to this myth. Inappropriate sexual behaviors
in people with dementing illnesses are uncommon. In a recent
study of our patients we found no instances of such behavior.

Accidental self-exposure and aimless masturbation do sometimes happen. Confused people may wander out in public
undressed or partially dressed simply because they have
forgotten where they are, how to dress, or the importance of
being dressed. They may undo their clothes or lift up a skirt
because they need to urinate and have forgotten where the
bathroom is. They may undress because they want to go to
bed or because a garment is uncomfortable.

Don't overreact to this. Just lead the person calmly back to his room or to the bathroom. If you find the person undressed, calmly bring him a robe and matter-of-factly help him put it on. The man who sat on the porch undressed had taken off his clothes because it was hot. He was unable to recognize that he was outside, was in sight of other people, and was not in the privacy of his home. Most confused people will never exhibit even this kind of behavior because their lifelong habits of modesty may remain.

Undressing or fidgeting with clothing can often be stopped by changing the kind of clothing the person wears. For example, use pants that pull on instead of pants with a fly in them. Use blouses that slip on or zip up the back instead of buttoning in front.

In our culture we have strong negative feelings about masturbation and such actions are upsetting to most families. Remember, this behavior, when it occurs, is a part of the brain damage. The person is only doing what feels good. He has forgotten his social manners. This does not mean that the person will develop other offensive sexual behaviors. If this occurs, try not to act upset, because it may precipitate a catastrophic reaction. Gently lead the person to a private place. Try distracting him by giving him something else to do. If a person's fidgeting is suggestive or embarrassing, also try giving him something else to do or something else to fidget with.

We know of no case in which a person with a dementing illness has exposed himself to a child and we do not wish to contribute to the myths about "dirty old men" by focusing on such behavior. However, should such an incident occur, react matter-of-factly and without creating any more fuss than is absolutely necessary. Your reaction may have much more impact on the child than the actual incident had. Remove the person quietly and explain to the child, "He forgets where he is."

We have observed that some people with dementing illnesses

have a diminished sex drive, and some have more interest in sex than they did previously. If a person develops increased sexuality, remember that, however distressing this is, it is a factor of the brain injury. It is not a factor of personality or a reflection on you or your marriage. (See p. 244.)

Don't hesitate to discuss upsetting sexual behavior with the doctor, a counselor, or even other families. They can help you understand and cope with it. The person you choose should be knowledgeable about dementia and comfortable discussing sexual matters. He may make specific suggestions to reduce the behavior. Also see Chapter 12: "Sexuality" and "Getting Help."

## CHANGING ANNOYING BEHAVIORS

Sometimes the little things that the impaired person does are what really get to you. You may have some success reducing or eliminating annoying behaviors with this method.

First, select *one* specific behavior that happens often and that you would really like to change. You will have most success with certain kinds of behaviors, such as repeating the same question over and over. Behaviors that arise out of catastrophic reactions are not easily changed by this method but are best managed by eliminating the precipitating cause. Next, get the cooperation of everyone in the household in your plan. This method works only if everyone participates. Finally, respond with warmth and affection to all the pleasant things the person does and *absolutely ignore* the selected annoying behavior. Do not try to argue with the person, scold him, or respond *in any way at all* to the annoying behavior. A negative response, such as scolding, can have the opposite effect from what you want, so that the person continues the behavior. This is not because he is obstinate (he can't remember long enough to do it deliberately) but because you have reminded him of his habit by calling his attention to it.

This system works best if you focus on one specific problem area at a time. It works only if everyone cooperates by *always* ignoring the behavior. It will not work if you occasionally respond to the behavior. This is why everyone in the house must participate. A vital part of the process is giving the person obvious attention when he behaves pleasantly. It may take several weeks of patient effort before you see a change.

This method worked for one husband who was particularly upset when his wife asked every night, "Who are you? What are you doing in my bed?" He stopped trying to explain to her and began simply ignoring the question. He would turn his head away slightly or turn his back on her and pretend she had not said anything. Eventually she stopped asking the question.

A similar method for changing annoying physical activities is to follow the same patterns except to respond to the behavior by distracting the person each time the behavior occurs. Again, do not scold the person for the behavior. For example,

*One woman was restless much of the time. She paced, fidgeted, and wandered. Her husband stopped telling her to sit down and instead began handing her a deck of cards, saying, "Here, Helen, play some solitaire." He took advantage of her lifelong enjoyment of this card game, even though she no longer played it correctly.*

## REPEATING THE QUESTION

Sometimes it is the little things that seem to be the last straw in living with a person with a dementing illness. Many families find that confused people ask the same question over and over and that this is extremely irritating. In part, this may be a symptom of the fear and insecurity of a person who can no longer make sense out of his surroundings. The person may not remember things for even brief periods, so he may have no recollection of having asked you before or of your answer. Try the technique described for changing annoying behaviors.

Sometimes, instead of answering the question again, it is helpful to reassure the person that everything is fine and that you will take care of things. Sometimes the person is really worried about something else, which he is unable to express. If you can correctly guess what this is and reassure him, he may relax. For example,

*Mr. Rockwell's mother kept asking, "When is my mother coming for me?" When Mr. Rockwell told her that her mother had been dead for many years, she would either get upset or ask the question again in a few minutes. Mr. Rockwell realized that the question really expressed her feelings that she was lost, and began responding by saying, "I will take care of you." This obviously calmed his mother.*

## REPETITIOUS ACTIONS

An occasional and distressing behavior that may occur in people with a brain disease is the tendency to repeat the same action over and over.

*Mrs. Weber's mother-in-law folded the laundry over and over. Mrs. Weber was glad the older woman was occupied, but this same activity upset her husband. He would shout, "Mother, you have already folded that towel five times."*

*Mrs. Andrews had trouble with baths. She would wash just one side of her face. "Wash the other side," her daughter would say, but she kept on washing the same spot.*

*Mr. Barnes paces around and around the kitchen in the same pattern, like a bear in a cage.*

150

It seems as if the damaged mind has a tendency to "get stuck" on one activity and has difficulty "shifting gears" to a new activity. When this happens, gently suggest that the person do a specific new task, but try not to pressure him or sound upset, because you can easily precipitate a catastrophic reaction.

In the case of Mrs. Weber's mother-in-law, ignoring the problem worked well. As Mr. Weber came to accept his mother's illness, the behavior ceased to bother him.

Mrs. Andrews's daughter found out that gently patting her mother's cheek where she wanted her to wash next would get her out of the repetitious pattern. In this example, a stroke had lessened her mother's awareness of one side of her body. Touch is a very good way to get a message to the brain when words fail. Touch the arm you want a person to put in a sleeve; touch the place you want the person to wash next; touch a hand with a spoon to get a person to pick it up.

Mr. Barnes's wife found ways to distract his pacing by giving him something to do. "Here, Joe, hold this," she would say, and hand him a spoon. "Now hold this," and she would take the spoon and give him a potholder. "Helping" would enable him to stop pacing. It kept him busy and perhaps also made him feel needed.

## CLINGING OR PERSISTENTLY FOLLOWING YOU AROUND

Families tell us that forgetful people sometimes follow them from room to room, becoming fretful if the care taker disappears into the bathroom or basement, or that they constantly interrupt whenever the care giver tries to rest or get a job done. This can be distressing. Few things can irritate more than being followed around all the time.

This behavior can be understood when we consider how strange the world must seem to a person who constantly forgets. The trusted care giver becomes the only security in a world of confusion. When one cannot depend on himself to remember the necessary things in life, one form of security is to stick close to someone who does know.

The memory-impaired person cannot remember that if you go in the bathroom, you will be right back out. To his mind, with his confused sense of time, it may seem as if you have vanished. Child-proof doorknobs on the bathroom door may help give you a few minutes of privacy. Sometimes setting a timer and saying "I will be back when the timer goes off" will help. One husband got himself a set of headphones so he could listen to music while his wife continued to talk. (Then he got her a set because he discovered that she enjoyed the music.)

It is most important that you try not to let annoying behaviors such as these wear you down. You must find other people who will help with the person so you can get away and do the things that relax you—go visiting or shopping, take a nap, or enjoy an uninterrupted bath.

Find simple tasks that the person can do, even if they are things that you could do better or things that are repetitious. Winding a ball of yarn, dusting, or stacking magazines may make a person feel useful and will keep him occupied while you do your work.

*Mrs. Hunter's mother-in-law, who has a dementing illness, followed Mrs. Hunter around the house never letting her out of her sight and always criticizing. Mrs. Hunter hit upon the idea of having her mother-in-law fold the wash. Since Mrs. Hunter has a large family, she has a lot of wash. The older woman folds, unfolds, and refolds (not very neatly) and feels like a useful part of the household.*

Is it being unkind to give a person made-up tasks to keep her occupied? Mrs. Hunter doesn't think so. The confused woman needs to feel that she is contributing to the family and she needs to be active.

## COMPLAINTS AND INSULTS

Sometimes people with dementing illnesses repeatedly complain, despite your kindest efforts. The confused person may say things like "You are cruel to me," "I want to go home," "You stole my things," or "I don't like you." When you are doing all that you can to help, you may feel hurt or angry when the confused person says such things. When he looks and sounds well or when such criticism comes from someone you have looked up to, your first response may be to take the criticism personally. You can quickly get into a painful and pointless argument, which may cause him to have a catastrophic reaction and perhaps even scream, cry, and throw things at you, leaving you exhausted and upset.

If this happens, step back and think through what is happening. Even though the person looks well, he actually has an injury to his brain. The experiences of having to be cared for, feeling lost, and losing possessions and independence may seem to the confused person like a cruel experience. "You are cruel to me" may really mean "life is cruel to me." Because the person cannot accurately sort out the reality around him, he may misinterpret your efforts to help as stealing from him. He may not be able to accept, understand, or remember the facts of his increasing impairment, his financial situation, the past relationship he had with you, and all of the other things you are aware of. For example, he knows only that his things are gone and you are there. Therefore, he feels that you must have stolen his things.

A family member contributed the following interpretations of the things her husband often said. Of course, we cannot know what a brain-impaired person feels or means, but this wife has found loving ways to interpret and accept the painful things her husband says.

*He says: "I want to go home."*
*He means: "I want to go back to the condition of life, the quality of life, when everything seemed to have a purpose and I was useful, when I could see the products of my hands, and when I was without the fear of small things."*

*He says: "I don't want to die."*
*He means: "I am sick although I feel no pain. Nobody realizes just how sick I am. I feel this way all of the time, so I must be going to die. I am afraid of dying."*

*He says: "I have no money."*
*He means: "I used to carry a wallet with some money in it. It is not in my back pants pocket now. I am angry because I cannot find it. There is something at the store that I want to buy. I'll have to look some more."*

*He says: "Where is everyone?"*
*He means: "I see people around me but I don't know who they are. These unfamiliar faces do not belong to my family. Where is my mother? Why has she left me?"*

In coping with remarks such as these, avoid contradicting the person or arguing with him; those responses may lead to a catastrophic reaction. Try not to say "I didn't steal your things," "You *are* home," "I gave you some money." Try not to reason with the person. Saying "Your mother died thirty years ago" will only confuse and upset him more.

Some families find it helpful to ignore many of these complaints or to use distractions. Some families respond sympathetically to the feeling they think is being expressed: "Yes, dear, I know you feel lost," "Life does seem cruel," "I know you want to go home."

Of course, you may get angry sometimes, especially when you have heard the same unfair complaint over and over. To do so is human. Probably the confused person will quickly forget the incident.

Sometimes the impaired person loses the ability to be tactful. He may say, "I don't like John," and you may know he never did like this person. This can be upsetting. It helps for those involved to understand that the person is unable to be tactful, that while he may be being honest he is not being purposefully unkind.

Perhaps you can cope with these remarks, but what about other people? Sometimes people with dementing illnesses make inappropriate or insulting remarks to other people. These can range from naïve directness, such as telling the pastor's wife she has a run in her stocking, to insults, such as shouting at the neighbor who brings dinner, "Get out of my house, you're trying to poison us."

Confused people may pick up things in a store and not pay for them, or may accuse the sales clerk of stealing their money. They may tell casual friends or strangers stories such as "My daughter keeps me locked in my room." When you take a confused person to visit he may put on his coat and say, "Let's go home. This place stinks."

Each brain-impaired person is different. Some will retain their social skills. In others a tendency toward bluntness may emerge as open rudeness. Some are fearful and suspicious, leading them to make accusations. Catastrophic reactions account for some of this behavior. The confused person often misjudges who the person is that he is speaking to or he misjudges the situation.

*A secretary was talking with a confused man while the doctor talked to his wife. He was obviously trying to make polite conversation, but he had lost the subtlety he once had. "How old are you?" he asked, "You look pretty old." When she answered another question that no, she was not married, he said, "I guess no one would have you."*

People chuckle at this sort of behavior in a small child because everyone understands that a child has not yet learned good manners. It will be helpful to you if most of the people around you understand that the person has a dementing illness that affects his memory of good manners. Dementing illnesses are common enough that as public awareness develops more people will recognize that these behaviors are the result of specific diseases and that, while such behavior is sad, it is not deliberate.

To those people who see you and the confused person often, such as neighbors, friends, church members, and perhaps familiar store clerks, you may want to give a brief explanation of the person's illness. When you make this explanation, you should reassure people that this illness does not make the person dangerous, and that the person is not crazy.

Should a confused person create a scene in a public place, perhaps due to a catastrophic reaction, remove him gently. It may be best to say nothing. While this can be embarrassing, you do not necessarily owe strangers any explanation.

Distraction is a good way to get a confused person out of what might become an embarrassing situation. For example, if he is asking personal questions, change the subject. When a person is telling others that you are keeping him prisoner or not feeding him, try distracting him. Avoid denying directly, as this can turn into an argument with the confused person. If these are people you know you may want to explain to them later. If they are strangers, ask yourself whether or not it really matters what strangers think.

If a person is taking things in stores, he may be doing so because he has forgotten to pay for them or because he does not realize that he is in a store. Several families have found that giving the person things to hold or asking him to push the shopping cart, so that his hands are occupied, will stop the problem. Before you leave the store, check to see if he has anything in his pockets. You may want to dress him in something that has no pockets the next time you go shopping.

Sometimes there is a gossip or insensitive person in a community who may build upon the inappropriate remarks of a person with a dementing illness. It is important that you not be upset by such gossip. Usually other people have an accurate estimate of the truth of such gossip.

## FORGETTING TELEPHONE CALLS

Forgetful people who can still talk clearly often continue to answer the telephone or to make calls. However, they may not remember to write down telephone messages. This can upset friends, confuse people, and cause you considerable inconvenience and embarrassment.

There are several inexpensive devices sold at electronics stores that will record all telephone conversations. Attaching the device to an extension phone the impaired person does not often use may be wise. With this taped record of calls, you can call people back, explain the situation, and respond to their call.

*One husband writes, "I found out from the tape that she called the dentist five times about her appointment. Since I knew about it I called them and told them how to manage that."*

In some areas the telephone company offers a "call-forwarding service," which will transfer calls to your home to another telephone number. You may want to check with the telephone company to find out under what circumstances it is legal to tape-record calls.

## DEMANDS

*Mr. Cooper refused to stop living alone, even though it was clear to his family that he could not manage. Instead, he called his daughter at least once a day with real emergencies that sent her dashing across town to help out. His daughter felt angry and manipulated. She was neglecting her own family, and she was exhausted. She felt that her father had always been a self-centered, demanding person, and that his current behavior was deliberately selfish.*

*Mrs. Dietz lived with her daughter. The two women had never gotten along well and now Mrs. Dietz had Alzheimer's disease. She was wearing her daughter out with demands: "Get me a cigarette," "Fix me some coffee." The daughter could not tell her mother to do these things herself because she started fires.*

Sometimes people with dementing illnesses can be demanding and appear to be self-centered. This is especially hard to accept when the person does not appear to be significantly impaired. If you feel that this is happening, try to step back and objectively evaluate the situation. Is this behavior deliberate or is it a symptom of the disease? The two can look very much alike, especially when the person had a way of making people feel manipulated before he developed a dementing brain disease. However, what is often happening with an impaired person is *not* something he can control. Manipulative behavior really requires the ability to plan, which the person with a dementing illness is losing. What you experience are old styles of relating to others which are no longer really deliberate. An evaluation can be helpful because it tells you objectively how much of such behavior is something the person can remember to do or not to do.

Some demanding behavior reflects the impaired person's feelings of loneliness, fright, or loss. For example, when a person has lost his ability to comprehend the passage of time and to remember things, being left alone for a short time can feel that he has been abandoned and he may accuse you of deserting him. Realizing that this behavior reflects such feelings can help you not to feel so angry and it can help you respond to the *real* problem (for example, that he feels abandoned) instead of responding to what seems to you like selfishness or manipulation.

Sometimes you can devise ways for the confused person to continue to feel a sense of control over his life and mastery over his circumstances which are not so demanding of you.

*Mr. Cooper's daughter was able to find an "apartment" for her father in a sheltered housing building where meals, social services, and housekeeping were provided. This reduced the number of emergencies but enabled Mr. Cooper to continue to feel independent.*

*A medical evaluation confirmed for Mrs. Dietz's daughter that her mother could not remember her previous requests for a cigarette for even five minutes. With the help of the physician, she was able to deal with her mother's addiction to cigarettes and coffee.*

Families often ask whether they should "spoil" the person by meeting his demands or whether they should try to "teach" him to behave differently. The best course may be neither of these. Since he cannot control his behavior, you are not "spoiling" him, but it may be impossible for you to meet endless demands. And since the impaired person has limited ability, if any, to learn, you cannot teach him and scolding may precipitate catastrophic reactions.

If the person demands that you do things you think he can do, be sure that he really can do these things. He may be overwhelmed by the tasks. Simplifying them may make him willing to do them. Sometimes being very specific and direct with the person helps. Saying "I am coming to see you Wednesday" is more helpful than getting into an argument over why you don't visit more often. Say "I will get you a cigarette when the timer goes off. Do not ask me for one until the timer goes off." Ignore further demands until then.

You may have to set limits on what you realistically can do. But before you set limits, you need to know the extent of the impaired person's disability and you need to know what other resources you can mobilize to replace what you cannot do. You may need to enlist the help of an outside person—a nurse or social worker who understands the disease—to help you work out a plan that provides good care for the sick person without leaving you exhausted or trapped.

When demands make you feel angry and frustrated, try to find an outlet for your anger which does not involve the impaired person. Your anger can precipitate catastrophic reactions, which may make him even more recalcitrant.

## WHEN THE SICK PERSON INSULTS THE SITTER

When a family is able to arrange for someone to stay with the impaired person, he may fire the sitter or housekeeper. He may get mad or suspicious, insult her, not let her in, or accuse her of stealing. This can make it seem impossible for you to get out of the house, or mean that the impaired person can no longer live in his own home. Often you can find ways to solve the problem.

As with many other problems, this situation may arise out of the impaired person's inability to make sense out of his surroundings or to remember explanations. All he may recognize is that a stranger is in the house. Sometimes the presence of a "babysitter" means a further loss of his independence, which he may realize and react to.

Make sure the sitter knows that it is you, not the confused person, who has the authority to hire and fire. This means that you must trust the sitter absolutely. If possible, find a sitter the person already knows or introduce the person to the sitter gradually. The first time or two, have the sitter come while you remain at home. Eventually the person may become accustomed to the idea that the sitter belongs there. This will also give you an opportunity to teach the sitter how you manage certain situations and to evaluate how well the sitter relates to the confused person.

Be sure the sitter understands the nature of a dementing illness and knows how behaviors such as catastrophic reactions are handled. (Hiring a sitter is discussed in Chapter 10.) Try to find sitters who are adept at engaging the person's trust and who are clever about managing the person without triggering a catastrophic reaction. Just as there are some people who are naturally good with children and others who are not, there are some people who are intuitively adept with confused people. However, they are often hard to find.

Be sure the sitter can reach you, another family member, or the doctor in the event of a problem.

Often the confused person will adjust to the presence of a sitter if both you and the sitter can weather the initial, stormy period.

# 8

## PROBLEMS OF MOOD

### DEPRESSION

PEOPLE WITH MEMORY PROBLEMS may also be sad, low, or depressed. When a person has memory problems and is depressed it is very important that a careful diagnosis be made and the depression treated. The memory problems may not be caused by Alzheimer's disease and may get better when the depression improves. The person may have both Alzheimer's disease and a depression that will respond to treatment.

When a person with an incurable disease is depressed, it can seem logical that she is depressed about the chronic illness. But not all people with Alzheimer's disease or other chronic illnesses are depressed. Some seem not to be aware of their problems. A certain amount of discouragement about one's condition is natural and understandable, but a deep despondency or a continuing depression is neither natural nor necessary. Fortunately, this kind of depression responds well to treatment, so the person can feel better whether or not she also has an irreversible dementing illness.

Researchers are trying to understand why we get depressed, but the total answer is not yet in. We obviously feel sad or low when something bad happens to us. But this does not completely explain the phenomenon of depression. For example, researchers are linking some depressions to changes in the brain. It is important that a physician assess the nature of each depression and determine whether it is a response to a situation or a deeper despondency, and then treat the depression appropriately. Indications of a deeper despondency include weight loss, a change in sleep patterns, feelings that one has done something bad and deserves to be punished, or a preoccupation with health problems.

It may be impossible for a depressed person to "snap out of it" by herself. Telling her to do so may only increase her feelings of frustration and discouragement. For some people, trying to cheer them makes them feel that they are not understood.

You can encourage a depressed or discouraged person to continue to be around other people. If she has memory problems, be sure that the activities she tries are things she can still do successfully and are of some use, so that she can feel good about herself for doing them. Help her avoid tasks that are too complicated. Even small failures can make her feel more discouraged about herself. Have her set the table for you. If she doesn't have that much energy, have her set just one place. If that task is too complicated, have her set out just the plates.

If groups of people upset her, encourage her not to withdraw completely but instead to talk with one familiar person at a time. Ask one friend to visit. Urge the friend to talk to the depressed person, to meet her eyes and involve her.

If the person often complains about health problems, it is

important to take these complaints seriously and have a doctor determine whether there is a physical basis for the complaints. (Remember that chronic complainers can get sick. It is easy to overlook real illnesses when a person often focuses on things with no physical basis.) When you and the doctor are sure that there is no physical illness present, he can treat the depression that is the underlying cause of the problem. Never let a physician dismiss a person as "just a hypochondriac." People who focus on health problems are really unhappy and need appropriate care.

## SUICIDE

When a person is depressed, demoralized, or discouraged, there is always a possibility that she will harm herself. While it may be difficult for a person with Alzheimer's disease to plan a suicide, you do need to be alert to the possibility that she will injure herself. If the person has access to a knife, a gun, power tools, solvents, medications, or car keys, she may use them to kill or maim herself.

## ALCOHOL OR DRUG ABUSE

Depressed people may use alcohol, tranquilizers, or other drugs to try to blot out the feelings of sadness. This can compound the problem. In a person with a dementing illness it can also further reduce her ability to function. You need to be especially alert to this possibility in a person who is living alone or who has used medications or alcohol in the past.

People who are heavy drinkers and who also develop a dementing illness can be difficult for their families to manage. The person may be more sensitive to small amounts of alcohol than a well person, so even one drink or one beer can significantly reduce her ability to function. These people often do not eat properly, causing nutritional problems that further impair them. They may also act nasty, stubborn, or hostile.

It helps to recognize that the brain impairment may make it impossible for the person to control her drinking or her other behaviors, and that you may have to provide this control for her. This will include taking steps to end her supply of alcohol. Do so quietly but firmly. Try not to feel that her unpleasant behavior is aimed at you personally. Avoid saying things that put the blame for the situation on anybody. Do what needs to be done, but try to find ways for the person to retain her self-esteem and dignity. There should be no liquor in the house unless it is locked away. One family was able to arrange with the local liquor store to stop selling to the patient.

You may need help from a counselor or physician to manage the behavior of a person with a memory problem who also abuses alcohol or drugs.

## APATHY, LISTLESSNESS

Sometimes people with brain diseases become apathetic and listless. They just sit and don't want to do anything. Such people may be easier to care for than people who are upset, but it is important not to overlook them.

As with depression, we are not sure why some people become apathetic and listless. However, it is important to keep them as active as possible. People need to move around and to use their minds and bodies as much as they can.

Withdrawing may be a person's way of coping when things get too complicated for her, and if you insist on her participation she may have a catastrophic reaction. Try to reinvolve her at a level at which she can feel comfortable, can succeed, and can feel useful. Ask her to do a simple task, take her for a walk and point out interesting things, play some music, or go for a car ride.

It often seems that getting the body moving helps cheer a person up. Once a person gets started doing something, she may begin to feel less apathetic. Perhaps she can peel only one potato today. Tomorrow she may feel like doing two. Perhaps she can spade the garden. Even if she spades for only a few minutes, it may have helped for her to get moving. If she stops a task after a few minutes, instead of urging her to go on, focus your attention on what she has accomplished and compliment her on that.

Occasionally, when you try to get a person active, she may become upset or agitated. If this happens, you will need to weigh the importance of her being active against her being upset.

## ANGER

Sometimes people with dementing illnesses become angry. They may lash out at you as you try to help them. They may slam things around, hit you, refuse to be cared for, throw food, yell, or make accusations. This can be upsetting for you and may cause problems in the household. It can seem as if all this hostility is aimed at you, despite your best efforts to take care of the person and you may be afraid that the person will hurt herself or someone else when she lashes out in anger. This is certainly a real concern. However, our experience has been that it actually occurs rarely and can usually be controlled.

*Angry or violent behavior is usually a catastrophic reaction and should be handled as you would any other catastrophic reaction.* Respond calmly; do not respond with anger. Remove the person from the situation or remove the upsetting stimulus. Look for the event that precipitated the reaction so that you can prevent or minimize a recurrence.

Try not to interpret anger in the same way as you would if it came from a well person. Anger from a confused person is often exaggerated or misdirected. The person may not really be angry at you at all. The anger is probably the result of misunderstanding what is happening. For example,

*Mr. Jones adored his small grandson. One day the grandchild tripped and fell and began to cry. Mr. Jones grabbed a knife, began to yell, and would allow no one near the child.*

*Mr. Jones had misinterpreted the cause of the child's crying and overreacted. He thought someone was attacking the child. Fortunately, the child's mother understood what was happening. "I will help you protect the baby," she said to Mr. Jones. She gave Mr. Jones a job to do: "Here, you hold the door for me." Then she was able to pick up and quiet the child.*

Forgetfulness is an advantage, since the person may quickly forget the episode. Often you can distract a person who is behaving this way by suggesting something you know she likes.

*Mrs. Williams's mother-in-law often got angry and nasty when Mrs. Williams tried to prepare supper. Mr. Williams began distracting his mother by spending that time each day visiting with just her in another part of the house.*

Once in a while a person experiencing a catastrophic reaction will hit someone who is trying to help her. Respond to this as you would to a catastrophic reaction. When at all possible, do not restrain her. If this occurs frequently you may need to ask the doctor to help you review what is upsetting the person and if necessary to consider prescribing medication.

## NERVOUSNESS AND RESTLESSNESS

People with dementing illnesses may become worried, anxious, agitated, and upset. They may pace or fidget. Their constant restlessness can get on your nerves. The person may not be able to tell you why she is upset. Or she may give you an unreasonable explanation for her anxiety. For example,

*Mrs. Berger was obviously upset over something, but whenever her husband tried to find out what it was, she would say that her mother was coming to get her. Telling her that her mother had been dead for years only caused her to cry.*

Some anxiety and nervousness may be caused by the changes within the brain. Other nervousness may come from real feelings of loss or tension. Even severely ill people remain sensitive to the moods of the people around them. If there is tension in the household, no matter how well you try to conceal it, the person may respond to it. For example, Mrs. Powell argued with her son over something minor, and just when that was solved, her confused mother began to cry because she "felt like something dreadful was going to happen." Her feeling was a real response to the mood in the house, but because she was cognitively impaired, her interpretation of the cause of the feeling was incorrect.

The person may be sad and worried over losing some specific item, like her watch. Reassuring her that you have the watch may not seem to help. Again, she has an accurate *feeling* (something is lost: her memory is lost, time is lost, many things are lost), but the *explanation* of the feeling is inaccurate. Respond with affection and reassurance to her feeling, which is real, and avoid trying to convince her that what she expresses is unreasonable.

Trying to get the person to explain what is troubling her or arguing with her ("there is no reason to get upset") may only make her more upset. For example,

*Every afternoon at 2:00, Mrs. Novak began to pace and wring her hands at the day care center. She told the staff*

*that she was going to miss the train to Baltimore. Telling her she was not going to Baltimore only upset her more. The staff realized that she was probably worried about going home, and they reassured her that they would see that she got home safely. This always calmed her down. (They had responded appropriately to her feelings.)*

Not all anxiety and nervousness may go away so easily. Sometimes these feelings are inexplicable. Offering the person comfort and reassurance and trying to simplify her environment may be all that you can do to counteract the effects of her brain disease.

When people with dementing illnesses pace, fiddle with things, resist care, shove the furniture around, run away from home or from the day care center, or turn on the stove and all the water faucets they may make others around them nervous. Their restless, irritable behavior is hard for families to manage without help.

Agitation may be a part of depression, anger or anxiety. It may be restlessness or boredom, a symptom of pain, caused by medications, or an inexplicable part of the dementing illness. Respond calmly and gently; try to simplify what is going on around the person, and avoid "overloading her mental circuits." Your calmness and gentleness will communicate to her.

You may find it helpful to give the person who is mildly restless something to fiddle with. Some people will play with worry beads or with pennies in their pockets. Giving the person something constructive to do with her energy, such as walking to the mailbox after the mail, may help. If the person is drinking caffeinated beverages (coffee, cola, tea), switching to noncaffeinated drinks might help.

Sometimes this behavior is the result of frequent or almost continuous catastrophic reactions. Try to find ways to reduce the confusion, extra stimulation, noise, and change around the confused person. (Read the sections on catastrophic reactions and on wandering.) Medications may help very agitated or restless people.

## FALSE IDEAS, SUSPICIOUSNESS, PARANOIA, AND HALLUCINATIONS

Forgetful people may become unreasonably suspicious. They may suspect or accuse others of stealing their money, their possessions, and even things nobody would take, like an old toothbrush. They may hoard or hide things. They may shout for help or call the police. An impaired person may begin accusing her spouse of infidelity.

People with dementing illness may develop unshakable ideas that things have been stolen from them or that people are going to harm them. Carried to an extreme, these ideas can make the person fearful and resistant to all attempts at care and help. Occasionally they develop distressing and strange ideas that they seem to remember and insist upon. They may insist that this is not where they live, that people who are dead are alive and are coming for them, or that someone who lives in the house is a stranger and perhaps dangerous. Occasionally a person will insist that his wife is not his wife—she is someone who looks like his wife, but is an impostor.

A person with a dementing illness may hear, see, feel, or smell things that are not there. Such hallucinations may terrify her (if she sees a strange man in the bedroom) or amuse her (if she sees a puppy on the bed).

These behaviors are upsetting for families because they are strange and frightening and because we associate them with insanity. They may never happen to your family member, but you should be aware of them in case you have to respond to such an experience. When they occur in the presence of a dementing illness, they are usually the result of the brain injury or a superimposed delirium (see p. 325) and are not symptoms of other mental illness.

## Misinterpretation

Sometimes these problems are due to the person's misinterpretation of what she sees and hears. If she sees poorly in the dark, she may misinterpret the moving curtains as a strange man. If she hears poorly, she may suspect conversations to be people talking about her. If she loses her shoes, she may misinterpret the loss as a theft.

Is the person seeing accurately in the dark or is she not hearing as well as she should? The cognitively impaired person must be seeing and hearing as well as possible because she may not realize her sensory limitations. Be sure her glasses and/or hearing aid are working well. If the room is dimly lit, see if improving the lighting helps. If the room is noisy or if sounds are muted, the person may need help identifying sounds. (See Chapter 6: "Hearing Problems.")

If you think the person is misinterpreting things, you may be able to help by explaining what she sees or hears. Say, for example, "That movement is the curtains" or "That tapping noise is the bush outside your window." This is different from directly disagreeing with her, which may cause her to have a catastrophic reaction. Avoid saying "There is no man in the bedroom" or "Nobody is trying to sneak in. Now go to sleep."

If the person does not hear well, it may help to include her in the conversation by addressing her directly rather than talking about her. Look directly at her. Some people read lips enough to supplement their hearing. You might say, "Dad, John says the weather has been terrible lately," or "Dad, John says the new grandchild is sitting up now." Never talk about someone in the third person, as if she weren't there, no matter how "out of it" you think she is. This is dehumanizing, and can understandably make a person angry. Ask other people not to do it.

Sometimes the impaired person's brain incorrectly interprets what her senses see or hear correctly. This is often what happens when a person becomes unrealistically suspicious. Sometimes you can help by giving the confused person accurate information or writing down reminders. You may have to repeat the same information frequently, since the person will tend to forget quickly what you say.

## Failure to Recognize People or Things (Agnosia)

People with dementing illnesses may lost the ability to recognize things or people, not because they have forgotten them or because their eyes are not working but because the brain is not able to put together information properly. This is called *agnosia,* from Latin words meaning "to not know." It can be a baffling symptom. For example,

> *Mrs. Kravitz said to her husband, "Who are you? What are you doing in my house?"*

This is not a problem of memory. Mrs. Kravitz had not forgotten her husband; in fact, she remembered him quite well, but her brain could not figure out who he was from what her eyes saw.

> *Mr. Clark insisted that this was not his house, although he had lived there many years.*

He had not forgotten his home, but, because his brain was not working right, the place did not look familiar.

You can help by giving the person other information. It may help to say "I guess it doesn't look familiar, but this is your house." Hearing your voice may help her remember who you are. Help her focus on one familiar detail. "Here is your chair. Sit in it. It *feels* familiar."

## *"You Are Not My Husband"*

Occasionally a person with a dementing illness will insist that her spouse is not her spouse or that her home is not her real home. She may insist that it looks just like her real house, but someone has taken the real one away and replaced it with a fake one. We do not understand exactly what is happening but we do know that this distressing symptom is a part of the brain damage.

Reassure the person, "I am your wife," but avoid arguing. Although this may seem heartbreaking, it is important for you to reassure yourself that it is not a rejection of you (the person *does* remember you.) It is just an inexplicable confusion of the damaged brain.

## "My Mother Is Coming for Me"

Someone with a dementing illness may forget that a person she once knew has died. She may say, "My mother is coming for me," or she may say that she has been visiting with her grandmother. Perhaps her memory of the person is stronger than her memory of the death. Perhaps in her mind the past has become the present.

Instead of either contradicting her or playing along with her, try responding to her general feelings of loss, if you feel that this is what she is expressing.

Sometimes people feel that this idea is "spooky" or that the impaired person is "seeing the dead." It is much more likely to be just another symptom like forgetfulness, wandering, or catastrophic reactions.

Perhaps you will decide that this issue is not worth the argument.

## Suspiciousness

If a person is suspicious or "paranoid," one must consider the possibility that her suspicions are founded on fact. Sometimes when a person is known to be unusually suspicious, real causes for her suspiciousness are overlooked. In fact, she might be being victimized, robbed, or harassed. However, some people with dementing illnesses do develop a suspiciousness that is inappropriate to the real situation.

Paranoia and suspiciousness are not really difficult to understand. We are all suspicious; it is necessary to our survival. The innate naiveté of the child is carefully replaced by a healthy suspicion. We are taught to be suspicious of strangers who offer us candy, door-to-door salesmen, and people with "shifty" eyes. Some of us were also taught as children to be suspicious of people of other races or religions. Some people have always been suspicious, others always trusting. A dementing illness may exaggerate these personality traits.

*Ms. Henderson returns to her office to find her purse missing. Two other purses have disappeared this week. She suspects that the new file clerk has stolen it.*

*As Mr. Starr comes out of a restaurant at night, three teenagers approach him and ask for change for the telephone. His heart pounds. He suspects that they plan to mug him.*

*Mrs. Bellotti called her friend three times to meet for lunch and each time the friend refused, giving the excuse that she had extra work. Mrs. Bellotti worries that her friend is avoiding her.*

Situations like these occur frequently. One difference between the response of a well person and that of a brain-impaired person is that the latter's ability to reason may become overwhelmed by the emotions the suspiciousness raises or her inability to make sense out of her world.

*Ms. Henderson searched for her purse and eventually remembered that she had left it in the cafeteria, where she found it being held for her at the cash register.*

The confused person lacks the ability to remember. Therefore, she will never find her purse and will continue to suspect the file clerk, as Ms. Henderson would have if she had not been able to remember where it was.

*Knowing that he is in a lighted, well-traveled area, Mr. Starr suppresses his panic and hands over fifteen cents to the three teenagers. They thank him and run to the phone.*

The confused person lacks the ability to assess her situation realistically and to control her panic. She often overreacts. Therefore, she might have screamed, the boys would have run, the police would have been called, etc.

*Mrs. Bellotti discussed her concerns with a mutual friend and learned that her friend had been sick and had gotten behind in her work and was always eating at her desk.*

The confused person lacks the ability to test out her suspicions against the opinions of others and then to evaluate them.

The person with the dementing illness who becomes "paranoid" has not gone crazy. She lives in a world in which each moment is starting over with no memory of the moments that went before, in which things disappear, explanations are forgotten, and conversations make no sense. In such a world it is easy to see how healthy suspiciousness can get out of hand. For example, the person with a dementing illness forgets that you carefully explained that you have hired a housekeeper. Lacking the information she needs to assess accurately what is going on, she makes exactly the same assumption we would if we found a strange person in the house—that she is a thief.

The first step in coping with excessive suspiciousness is to understand that this is not behavior the person can control.

Second, it only makes things worse to confront the person or to argue about the truthfulness of the complaint. Avoid saying "I told you twenty times I put your things in the attic. Nobody stole them." Perhaps you can make a list of where things are: "Love seat given to cousin Mary. Cedar chest in Ann's attic."

When she says, "You stole my dentures," don't say "Nobody stole your teeth, you lost them again." Instead, say "I'll help you find them." Locating the lost article will often solve the problem. Articles that are mislaid seem stolen to the person who cannot remember where she put them and who cannot reason that nobody would want her dentures.

One son securely fastened a key to the bulletin board (so his mother could not remove and hide it). Every time she accused him of stealing her furniture, he replied gently, "All your things are locked in the attic. Here is your key to the attic where they all are."

Sometimes you can distract a person from her focus on suspiciousness. Look for the lost articles; try going for a ride or getting her involved in a task. Sometimes you can look for the real cause of her complaints and respond with sympathy and reassurance to her feelings of loss and confusion.

When many of a person's possessions must be disposed of so she can move into someone's home or a nursing home, she may insist that they have been stolen. When you have assumed control over a person's finances, she may accuse you of stealing from her. Repeated explanations or lists sometimes help. Often they do not, because the person cannot make sense out of the explanation or will forget it. Such accusations can be discouraging when you are doing the best you can for someone. These accusations are often, at least in part, an expression of the person's overwhelming feelings of loss, confusion, and distress. They are not really harmful to anyone, except that they are distressing for you. When you understand that they occur because of the brain damage, you will be less upset by them.

Few things make us more angry than being falsely accused. Consequently, the impaired person's accusations can alienate sitters, other family members, neighbors, and friends, causing you to lose needed sources of friendship and help. Make it clear to people that you do not suspect them of anything and explain to them that accusatory behavior results from the confused person's inability to assess reality accurately. Your trust in them must be obvious and strong enough to override the accusations made by the impaired person. Sometimes it is helpful to share with others written materials such as this book, which explain how the brain impairment affects behavior. Part of the problem is that the confused person may look and sound reasonable. She may not look and sound as if this behavior were beyond her control, and, because dementing illnesses are often poorly understood, people may not realize what is happening.

## Hiding Things

In a world that is confusing and in which things inexplicably disappear, it is understandable that a person would put things of importance in a safe place. The difference between being well and being impaired is that the impaired person forgets where that safe place is more often than the well person. Hiding behaviors often accompany suspiciousness, but because they cause so many problems of their own, we have discussed them separately in Chapter 7.

## Delusions and Hallucinations

Delusions are untrue ideas unshakably held by one person. They may be suspicious in nature ("The mafia are after me," or "You have stolen my money") or self-blaming ("I am a bad person,'' or ''I am rotting inside and spreading a terrible disease''). The nature of the delusion can help doctors diagnose the person's problem. Self-blaming ideas, for example, are often seen in people who are severely depressed. However, when delusions occur in a person who is known to have a brain impairment from strokes, Alzheimer's disease, or other conditions, the delusion is believed to arise out of the injury to brain tissue. It can be frustrating to have a person seem able to remember a false idea and unable to remember real information.

Sometimes delusions appear to come from misinterpreting reality. Sometimes they are tied to the person's past experiences. (A note of caution: not all odd things older people say are delusions.)

Hallucinations are sensory experiences that are real to the person having them but that others do not experience. Hearing voices or seeing things are most common, although occasionally people feel, smell, or taste things also.

*Mrs. Singer sometimes saw a dog asleep in her bed. She would call her daughter to ''come and get the dog out of my bed.''*

*Mr. Davis saw tiny little men on the floor. They distracted him, and often he sat watching them instead of taking part in activities at the senior center.*

*Mrs. Eckman heard burglars outside her window trying to break in and discussing how they would hurt her. She called the police several times and earned herself the reputation of a ''nut.''*

*Mr. Vaughan tasted poison in all his food. He refused to eat and lost so much weight that he had to be hospitalized.*

Hallucinations are a symptom, like a fever or sore throat, which can arise from many causes. Certain drugs can induce hallucinations in otherwise well people. Several disease processes can produce hallucinations. Just as with a fever or sore throat, the first step is to identify the cause of the hallucination. In an elderly person hallucinations are not necessarily an indication of a dementing illness. They may result from several causes, many of which are treatable. Delirium is one example. If hallucinations or delusions appear in a person who has previously been functioning well, they are probably not associated with dementia. Do not let a doctor dismiss this symptom as "senility." The examples we have given are not all examples of people in whom the hallucination is a symptom of dementia.

When hallucinations do develop as an inexplicable part of the dementing illness, your doctor can help. Often these symptoms respond to medications that make the patient more comfortable and life easier for you.

When delusions or hallucinations occur, react calmly so that you do not further upset the confused person. Although this is not an emergency situation, you will want to check with the doctor as soon as is convenient. Reassure the person that you are taking care of things and that you will see that things are all right.

Avoid denying the person's experience or directly confronting her or arguing with her. This will only further upset her. Remember, the experience is real for her. At the same time you should not play along with a delusion or a hallucination. You don't have to agree or disagree; just listen or give a noncommittal answer. You can say "I don't hear the voices you hear, but it must be frightening for you." This is not the same as agreeing with the person. Sometimes you can distract the person so that she forgets her hallucination. Say "Let's go in the kitchen and have a cup of warm milk." When she returns to her bedroom, she may no longer see a dog in her bed and you will have avoided an upsetting confrontation.

It is often comforting to touch the person physically, as long as she does not misinterpret your touch as an effort to restrain her. Say "I know you are so upset. Would it help if I held your hand (or gave you a hug)?"

# 9

## SPECIAL ARRANGEMENTS
## IF YOU BECOME ILL

ANYONE CAN BECOME ILL or suffer an accident. If you are tired and under stress from caring for a chronically ill person, your risk of illness or accident increases. The spouse of a person with a dementing illness, himself no longer young, is at risk of developing other illnesses.

What happens to the confused, forgetful person if you, the care giver, are injured or become ill? It is important that you have a plan ready. Perhaps you will never need to put your plan into effect, but because dementia disables a person in such a way that he cannot act in his best interests, you must make advance plans that protect you and the impaired person.

You need a physician who is familiar with your health to whom you can turn if you become ill, and who is available quickly in a crisis. In addition, you need to plan in advance for several kinds of possible problems: the sudden, severe problems that would arise if you had a heart attack or stroke or fell and broke a bone; the less sudden problems that would arise if you had a long illness, hospitalization, or surgery; and the problems that would arise if you got the flu or were at home, sick, for a few days.

*Mrs. Brady suddenly began having chest pains and knew she should lie quietly. She told her confused husband to go get their neighbor but he kept pulling at her arm and shouting. When she finally was able to telephone for help, he refused to let the ambulance attendants in the house.*

Even when an impaired person appears to function well he may become upset and unable to do things he usually can do. Should you suddenly become ill and unable to summon help yourself, the upset and confused person may not be able to summon help for you. He may misinterpret what is happening and impede efforts to get help.

There are several possible ways you can plan to summon help. If your area has an emergency telephone number (such as 911), try to teach the person to call for help. Post the number over the phone. Or, post the number of a relative who lives nearby and who will respond to a confused telephone call. Some telephone companies offer an automatic dialing service. With this device the telephone will automatically dial a prerecorded number of your choice if you or the confused person is able to dial one or two digits. You can paint this digit red with fingernail polish so that it is easily identified.

At least one company manufactures a "panic button" that you can carry with you. It is about the size of a pocket calculator. If you press the button on it, it will activate the automatic dial described above and send a prerecorded message. Such equipment is expensive, but in some situations it might be life-saving.

If you live near someone who is willing to respond in a crisis, you may be able to use fairly inexpensive walkie-talkies or intercoms to summon help. Inexpensive walkie-talkies are sold as toys. More sophisticated ones are used by police and security departments. One can be left in place in the responder's home and adapted to operate on house current so that it is always "on," ready to receive a signal. You carry the other with you. These will send a signal over a limited distance (one-half mile). More expensive versions have a longer range (several miles). You may need an F.C.C. license for equipment with a long range.

Many areas have programs for senior citizens in which someone will call once a day to see if you are all right. This may mean a long delay in getting help, but it is better than nothing.

Be sure that the person who would respond in a crisis has a key to your house. The upset, confused person may refuse to let anyone in.

If you must go into the hospital or if you are at home sick, you will want to plan carefully in advance for the care of the confused person. Changes are upsetting for them, and it is helpful to minimize changes as much as possible. The substitute care giver should be someone the person knows and someone who knows your routines for managing him. Be sure that the names and phone numbers of your doctor, the patient's doctor, the pharmacist, your lawyer, and close family members are written down where the person helping out in an emergency can find them.

Some families have made up a "cope notebook" in which they have jotted down the things another person would need to know, for example. "Dr. Brown (824-8787). John gets a pink pill one hour before lunch. He will take it best with orange juice. The stove won't work unless you turn on the switch that is hidden behind the toaster. John starts to wander around suppertime. You need to watch him then."

## IN THE EVENT OF YOUR DEATH

When someone close to you has a dementing illness, you have a special responsibility to provide for him if you should

185

die. Probably your plans will never have to be put into action, but they must, for the sake of the sick person, be made.

When a family member is unable to take care of himself, it is important that you have a will that provides for his care. Find a lawyer whom you trust, and have him draw up a will and any other necessary legal papers. Every state has a law that determines how property will be divided among your heirs if you do not make a will or if your will is not valid. However, this may not be the way you wanted your estate to be distributed. In addition to the usual matters of disposing of property to one's heirs, the following questions must be addressed, and appropriate arrangements made. (See Chapter 15.)

What arrangements have been made for your funeral, and who will carry these out? You can select a funeral director in advance and agree with him, in writing, what kind of funeral you will have and how much it will cost. Far from being macabre, this is a considerate and responsible act that ensures that things will be done as you wish and that saves your distraught family from having to do this in the midst of their grief. Funerals can be expensive, and advance plans make it possible for you to see that your money is spent as you wish.

What immediate arrangements have been made for care of the person with a dementing illness, and who will be responsible for seeing that they are carried out? Someone must be available immediately who will be kind and caring.

Do the people who will be caring for the person with a dementing illness know his diagnosis and his doctor, and do they know as much as possible of what you know about how to make him comfortable?

What financial provisions have been made for the person with a dementing illness, and who will administer them? If he cannot manage his own affairs, someone must be available with the authority to care for him. You will want to select a person whom you trust to do this rather than leave such an important decision to a court or judge.

Sometimes a husband or wife cares for years for a spouse with a dementing illness and does not want to burden sons or daughters with the knowledge of this illness.

*Said a daughter, "I had no idea anything was wrong with Mom because Dad covered for her so well. Then he had a heart attack and we found her like this. Now I have the shock of his death and her illness all at one time. It would have been so much easier if he had told us about it long ago. And we didn't know anything about dementia. We had to find out all the things he had already learned, and at such a difficult time for us."*

All members of the family need to know what is wrong with the impaired person and what plans have been made. An experience like this is one example of the disservice of "protecting" other members of the family.

You should have a succinct summary of your assets available for the person who will take over. This should include information on the location of wills, deeds, stocks, cemetery lot deeds, and information about the care of the confused person.

# 10

## GETTING OUTSIDE HELP

THROUGHOUT THIS BOOK we have emphasized the importance of finding time for yourself away from the responsibilities of caring for the impaired person. You may also need other kinds of help: someone to see that a person who is alone during the day gets her meals; someone to help give the person a bath; someone to watch the person while you shop, rest, or take a break; someone to help with the housework; or someone with whom you can talk things over. Some of this help can come from family members, friends, or neighbors.

Sometimes a neighbor will look in on the confused person; the druggist will keep track of prescriptions for you; the minister will listen when you are discouraged; a friend will sit with the person in an emergency; and so forth. As you plan, you should consider these resources because they are important to you. However, at some point most families look for outside help in obtaining information, making decisions, and planning for the long-term care of their afflicted family member. Many families find the help they need and manage effectively without extensive professional assistance. However, the burdens of caring for a demented person can be enormous.

Sometimes people have mixed feelings about seeking assistance. At the same time that you know you need help, you may feel that another person will not do the job as well as you, or you may find that changes upset the confused person. You may worry about the cost of help.

The decision to help should be shared by all involved members of the family. It is not unusual for differences of opinion to arise. Fewer misunderstandings develop when everyone is kept informed about what resources are available, what they cost, and what services they offer. When you seek help, you will need to think about what kind of help is right for you and the confused person. For example, it may be more difficult to find help for a person who is combative or who wanders. You may need to work with your doctor to reduce these behaviors in order to get the assistance you need.

There are a variety of individuals, local agencies, and national organizations which can offer help. These may be private or public, sectarian or nonsectarian, municipal, state, or federal. The process of finding these resources on your own can be long and tedious. The first contacts you make may not provide the needed information or assistance, or the ideal resources may not be available. You may be brushed off by busy staff. A social worker can be helpful to you. She knows how to get around these problems and locate the best available help for you. She also knows how to assess your needs and match them with the resources available in the community. (See Chapter 2.)

## LOCATING RESOURCES YOURSELF

If you do not have available the skills of a social worker, here are some suggestions on how to locate outside resources on your own.

## Getting Outside Help

When you begin to look for help, know what kind of help you need and what you want to know. Writing down your questions may help you organize them. It may be helpful to keep a notebook. List the potential places you can look for help, what they can do, and their cost, advantages, and drawbacks. Add to them as you learn of others. For example,

*Mrs. Connors wrote:*

| Needs | Ideas | Pros | Cons |
|---|---|---|---|
| Someone to stay with Bill when I shop. | Aunt Mary | She is willing, no cost. | She is critical of me. |
| | senior day care | Good care. Nice people. Gets him out and active. | Cost. He gets upset if I take him there. |
| | call Senior Center Hotline | (talked to Mrs. Jones, 877-3708, who suggested I call Welfare Dept.) | |
| | Welfare Dept. (877-9292) Mrs. Smith | Program not available to people with dementia. | |

It is also useful to take notes on your conversation, including the name of the person you speak with. (Don't hesitate to ask people to spell their names.) If you speak with someone else in the organization for more detailed information, it can be helpful to have a record of your prior contacts. This will help you keep information straight. Don't be ashamed or afraid to call back if you didn't understand the first time. Sometimes the person to whom you first speak will be unable to answer your questions.

Always ask to speak to someone who can answer your questions. The supervisor should be able to answer your questions or direct you to someone else who can. It may take you many phone calls and personal contacts before you reach someone who can offer the kind of help you need. It is important to keep looking and keep asking questions until you find some person or organization who can offer the help you need.

Even when an agency cannot provide the needed help, ask them to direct you to some other person or agency who may be able to help. Be patient but be persistent.

Sometimes you may not find what you need, even after a long and tiring search. Don't get discouraged about yourself if there is no help. The quality and quantity of available services vary from area to area.

Unfortunately, the needed resources for families of people with dementing illnesses may not be available: some agencies have a waiting list, or they will only take certain kinds of people, while other agencies may be too expensive. Inadequate resources and services are major problems that can be changed only through public recognition of the dementing diseases and the needs of families. It is not your fault if you cannot locate a service that is not available.

Perhaps you will want to accept what resources are available, even if they are not ideal, since you may find that obtaining even some help is better than trying to cope alone.

## KINDS OF SERVICES

Not all people who have dementing illnesses are elderly. However, there are additional resources for patients sixty or over. Most local offices on aging have a list of free or reduced-fee programs for people over sixty or over sixty-five. Many of these programs state that they serve only people over a certain age. However, you should know that the spouse of a person who qualifies by age may also qualify, and that many of these programs are required by law to serve the elderly *and* the handicapped. Younger people with dementing illnesses may be eligible. Ask.

Some programs serve only those people who have rehabilitative potential, that is, people who can be "cured." This may be required by their funding source. People who have had strokes or who have a depressive illness may qualify, while people who have been diagnosed as having Alzheimer's disease or who are described as "senile" do not. We believe that this is a discriminatory practice that will eventually change. Communities and policy makers must be educated to the facts that these are diseases and not old age, that aiding families is both fiscally sound and humane, and that funding for only rehabilitation is discriminatory.

The rising cost of nursing home care is leading policy makers to look at various alternatives to institutionalization, including day care and help at home. Some programs are designed to rehabilitate employable adults or children. Sometimes such a program will pay for glasses, hearing aids, or speech rehabilitation if it can be shown that this will improve a person's functioning (not necessarily reverse her disease). Under antidiscrimination laws these programs will occasionally help people with dementing illnesses.

Many of the senior citizen programs will not directly help the person with a chronic dementing illness, but they may help you. For example,

> *Mr. Harrigan was eligible for a free senior citizen pass to the college swimming pool. His daughter stayed with Mrs. Harrigan while he swam two evenings a week. This got Mr. Harrigan out of the house without making further demands on his limited income.*

State and national park user fees, fishing license fees, and fees for the use of recreation facilities are often reduced or waived for senior citizens. There are also senior centers and clubs that may offer a range of activities.

Many businesses offer discounts to senior citizens.

Many areas offer some free transportation service. This can be valuable if you do not drive.

There are various income and property tax breaks for older people which may save you money.

Some areas offer services such as dental care, discounted dentures, less expensive eyeglasses, legal counseling, social work help, referral services, and free tax assistance to people over sixty, their spouses, and the handicapped. Some programs provide prescription medications or appliances at reduced cost.

Some programs will repair older people's homes for reduced rates. You may be able to use such a program to install wheelchair ramps, locks, grab bars, and other safety devices.

In some areas, programs such as Meals-on-Wheels will bring a daily hot meal to people who cannot get out. These meals are often delivered by friendly, dedicated volunteers who will also check to see how a person living alone is doing, but they provide limited help for a person who is becoming confused and are no substitute for supervision.

There are many senior citizen volunteer service programs. Some may provide help for you. Others may provide a way for you and the forgetful person to remain active and spend time with other people. For example,

*Mr. Gillis had always been active. Now he had a mild dementia. Unable to continue his job, he was bored and restless. His daughter arranged for him to work as a senior citizen volunteer at a nearby nursing home, where he spaded gardens and weeded flowerbeds. He felt active and useful and the nursing home staff was able to remind him frequently what to do next.*

Food stamps, Medicaid, or Supplemental Security Income (S.S.I.) is available to some families who are on a limited income.

There are many other programs; we have referred to some of them in other parts of this book. You should find out just what is available in your area even if you don't feel you need the service now.

## HELP FROM FRIENDS AND NEIGHBORS

Often friends and neighbors offer to help you care for the confused person. How much help should you accept or ask for from friends and neighbors? Most people like to help, yet making too many demands on some may eventually cause them to pull away.

When you turn to friends and neighbors for help, there are several things you can do to help them feel comfortable helping you. Because dementing illnesses are unfamiliar to many people, those who help you need to understand why the sick person acts as she does. Offer information about the ill person's condition.

Some people are uncomfortable around those who are visibly upset. You may not want to express all of your distress to such people. Close friends may be more willing to share some of the emotional burden with you than people who do not know you well.

When you ask people to help you, give them enough advance notice, if possible, so that they can plan the time to help you. Remember to thank them, and avoid criticizing what they have done if their efforts are less than perfect.

Look for things others can do to help which they will not consider to be inconvenient. For example, neighbors may not mind "looking in" since they live close by, while more distant friends might resent being asked to make a long drive.

Suggest things a helper can do which he will feel are useful or productive and which he can do without upsetting the confused person or precipitating a catastrophic reaction.

## HAVING SOMEONE COME INTO YOUR HOME

Many families can continue to care for a person if they are able to arrange for someone to come into their home to help. Such a person may be another family member, friend, neighbor, church member, paid or volunteer visitor, hired housekeeper, or nurse. Unfortunately, resources for help at home are limited, may not be available, or may be expensive. When they are available, care providers may be reluctant to serve the so-called senile. A social worker can help you utilize what is available.

It is important that helpers understand the nature of the person's disability and that they know how to avoid or respond to catastrophic reactions. Helpers need to know how to reach you or another responsible family member in case of an emergency. Be sure the helper knows from *you* what the person can or cannot do and what special care he needs. Remember that the impaired person might give the helper misleading information.

If the sick person has complicating health problems, such as a heart or respiratory condition, a tendency to choke or fall, or seizures, you must carefully consider the skills of the person with whom you leave him. If the person gets upset easily you may need to discuss with the doctor ways to reduce these behaviors. We have discussed the problems that arise when the confused person rejects the visiting care giver on p. 160.

Church groups will sometimes organize a team of helpers. Sometimes they will bring in meals for a short period (for example, while you are sick).

Some people are able to find a person who will sit with the

impaired person part of the day and who may even prepare meals. Older women who need to work but who do not have formal work skills are a good source of such help.

Good people are often found through word of mouth. Ask your friends if they know of someone. One woman who does this sort of work may be able to recruit her friends. Sometimes a person can be found by advertising in the newspaper. Sometimes college students can be found through the student employment office of the local college.

*One high school student, instead of babysitting, stayed with a demented lady when her family went out for the evening. The confused woman wandered around the house, but as long as the student played hymns on the piano, the woman was quiet.*

Some students are gentle and kind, have had experience with their own grandparents, and are looking for work.

Obviously, as with anyone you are taking into your home, you should check a person's references and be sure that she understands the person's condition and is willing to care for a confused person. Have the person come into your home several times while you are there before you leave the person in her care. This helps the forgetful person get used to the presence of another person in the house.

Discuss fees and exact responsibilities before you hire anyone. Costs vary widely, but are generally higher in metropolitan areas.

It is unreasonable to expect a woman to clean and watch an ill person for the same salary she would be paid for housecleaning. Realistically, a domestic helper probably cannot look after the confused person and clean the house. It is challenging for you to do both and often impossible for someone unfamiliar with your home and with the impaired person. You may have to settle for a sitter and not a clean house.

Occasionally families are able to exchange services. Plans can be simple or elaborate; basically, two or three families agree to take turns sitting. You may sit with two confused people in your home for one afternoon a week. Then the next week someone else will sit, while you get an afternoon out. This works best when the impaired people are not agitated and do not wander. Such people enjoy the contact with others. The "rules" of exchange services should be clearly spelled out.

An organization of families might want to train one or two people in the management of people with a dementing illness. Such a person would have a full-time job dividing her time among several families.

Visiting Nurse Associations and home health agencies send professionals, nurses, social workers, and other therapists into homes to provide evaluation and care. A nurse, for example, may monitor the patient's status, change a catheter, bathe an ill person, and give injections. A speech therapist may help a stroke patient regain language skills, or a physical therapist may exercise the patient. Home health aides can help with personal care, meals, or shopping. These services may be covered by medical insurance. Medicare may cover such services if they are ordered by a physician. Medicare's allowable services are limited and may not be a resource to you. A licensed practical nurse can bathe patients, change beds, give breakfast, etc., but may not be covered by Medicare unless the person also requires skilled nursing care at least for periodic reassessment. This is important: if periodic nursing assessment is part of the needed care, Medicare may pay for the help of a home health aide.

Medicare regulations change with changes in federal policy and can be confusing to interpret. Ask the social worker or service provider agency to help you find out whether their services to you are reimbursable. It may be worthwhile to request that a decision be reviewed as it applies to your particular case, and for your local volunteer association to urge that regulations be interpreted so that these services are reimbursed for dementia patients.

Medicaid may pay for home care if the patient requires skilled care and is eligible for Medicaid.

Home health aides are sometimes available at low cost to low-income families on a limited basis. Check with the local department of social service. Some service agencies will pay part of the cost of a home health aide. Or if you are not eligible for financial help, you can pay the full cost of home health care from a private agency.

## CARE OUTSIDE YOUR HOME

Another way for you to obtain help with the care of a person with a dementing illness is to arrange for him to stay outside your home part of the time. There are several potential resources, one or more of which may be available in your community. A social worker, the Office on Aging, or the Health Department may be your best source of information. As with in-home resources, care providers outside the home are often reluctant to accept people with dementing illnesses and you may have to help them learn how to care for such people.

It is not unusual for a family to be discouraged by the first visit to a day care center or nursing home.

*Mr. Wilson said, "I went to see the day care center. The hospital told me this was an excellent center. But I can't put Alice in there. Those people are old and sick. One of them was dragging a shopping bag around and mumbling. One was drooling. Some of them were in these chairs with a tray across them, hanging on the tray or sleeping."*

The sight of other disabled or elderly people can be distressing, and our perception of a person we love is colored by our memory of how she used to be.

You may feel that such a program does not offer the individualized care that you can give at home. However, we have observed that getting out of the house and being with other people is good for the forgetful person. She may feel comfortable in a setting that does not demand much of her and may make friends with other impaired people.

If you find yourself reacting this way to places you visit, you may find it helpful to talk to other families who are already using the program. They can tell you how they felt, what places they found that they like, and how they have been able to accept things that upset them at first. You may need to weigh the importance of respite for yourself and the benefits of the impaired person's being with others against this concern.

The change to a new setting may upset the confused person; you may need to introduce her gradually and be prepared for an adjustment period. (See Chapter 4: "Moving.")

## Kinds of Settings

Expanded nutrition programs offer a hot lunch and a recreation program in a sheltered group setting for several hours each weekday. They usually do not provide medical care, give medicines, or take wandering, disruptive, or incontinent people. They are often staffed by lay or paraprofessional people and can be helpful for the mildly or moderately confused individual.

Nutrition programs are funded through the Older Americans Act, and serve people over sixty and their spouse. You can find them by calling your commission on aging. Some hot lunch programs are intended for the well elderly and an impaired person will not fit in. Other programs under the same or similar funding offer services to the "frail" elderly. You may be able to attend with your spouse if you wish.

Adult day care programs offer several hours a day of

structured recreation for people with limited abilities. They provide mental stimulation within the capabilities of a confused person. People frequently seem to enjoy life more, sleep better, and are more manageable at home once they are established in a day care program. We believe they are among the most important resources for families.

Adult day care centers vary in staff, services offered, and clients accepted. Requirements for licensing vary with each state. Some centers may not be licensed or under state supervision.

Fees for day care programs vary, often depending on the sources of federal or state funding they use. Some have sliding fee scales based upon your income or the client's income. Programs may be in connection with state or federal hospitals, nursing homes, mental health centers, churches, psychiatric facilities, or family service agencies. Some centers have a nurse or social worker on duty.

It can be difficult to find adequate day care centers for people with dementia. Some centers are not equipped to care for people who wander or to accommodate people who cannot climb stairs. Some programs can accept only people over sixty or over sixty-five. Some centers specialize in stroke patients, elderly alcoholics, and other individuals designated as "potentially rehabilitatable." Sometimes a professional (the doctor, nurse, or social worker) can help you if a center is reluctant to accept a person with a dementing illness.

Day hospitals offer medical services, recreation therapy, and occupational therapy for impaired people who live at home. They are staffed by nurses, social workers, physicians, and other professionals. Funding sources for day hospitals sometimes restrict admission to patients with rehabilitative potential. The time a person may stay in the day hospital is usually limited to the period of evaluation and treatment.

# 11

## YOU AND THE IMPAIRED PERSON AS PART OF A FAMILY

CHAPTERS 2–10 have discussed how to get help for the sick person and ways to care for him. However, you and your family are important also. A chronic dementing illness places a heavy burden on families: it may mean a lot of work or financial sacrifices; it may mean accepting the reality that someone you love will never be the same again; it continues on and on; it may mean that responsibilities and relationships within the family will change; it may mean disagreements within the family; it may mean that you feel overwhelmed, discouraged, isolated, angry, or depressed. You and the person with a dementing illness, as well as the other people close to him, all interact as part of a family system. This system can be severely stressed by a dementing illness. It is helpful to consider the changes that may occur in families that are faced with a chronic illness and to identify the feelings you may experience. Sometimes just knowing that what is happening to you has happened to others can make life easier. Often recognizing what is happening suggests ways to improve things.

It is important to know that almost all families do care for their elderly and sick as long as possible. It is simply not true that most Americans abandon their elderly or "dump" them into nursing homes. Studies have shown that although many older people do not live with their children, they are closely involved with or cared for by them. Families usually do all they can, often at great personal sacrifice, to care for ill elderly members before seeking help. Of course, there are families who do not care for ill family members. There are some who, because of illness or other problems, are unable to care for their elderly; there are a few who do not wish to; there are some elderly people who have no family to help them. But in the majority of cases, families are struggling to do the best they can for their ill elderly.

Most family members discover a closeness and cooperation as they work together to care for someone with a dementing illness. Sometimes, however, the pressures of caring for an ill person create conflicts in families or cause old disagreements to flare up. For example.

> Mr. Higgins said, "We can't agree on what to do. I want to keep Mother at home. My sister wants her in a nursing home. We don't even agree on what is wrong."

> Mrs. Tate said, "My brother doesn't call and he refuses even to talk about it. I have to take care of Mother alone."

In addition, the burden of caring for a person with a dementing illness can be exhausting and distressing for you.

> Mrs. Fried said, "I get so depressed. I cry. Then I lie awake at night and worry. I feel so helpless."

Watching someone close to you decline can be a painful experience. This chapter discusses some of the problems that arise in families, and Chapter 12 will discuss some of the feelings you may have.

It is important to remember that not all of your experiences will be unhappy ones. Many people feel a sense of pride in learning to cope with difficult situations. Many family members rediscover one another as they work together to care for an ill person. As you help a forgetful person enjoy the world around him, you may experience a renewed delight in sharing little things—playing with a puppy or enjoying flowers. You may discover a new faith in yourself, in others, or in God. Most dementing illnesses progress slowly, so you and your family member can look forward to many good years.

> *Mrs. Morales said, "Although it has been hard, it's been good for me in a lot of ways. It's given me confidence to know that I can manage things my husband always took care of, and in some ways my children and I have grown closer as he has gotten sick."*

Since this book is designed to help you with problems when they do occur, most of what we discuss are unhappy feelings and problems. We know that this is a one-sided view that reflects only part of what life is like for you.

The feelings and problems you and your family experience interact and affect one another. However, for simplicity, we have organized them into separate topics: changes in roles within the family, finding ways to cope with changes in roles and the family conflict that can arise, your own feelings, and finding ways to care for yourself.

## CHANGES IN ROLES

Roles, responsibilities, and expectations within the family change when one person becomes ill. For example,

> *A wife said, "The worst part is doing the checkbook. We have been married thirty-five years and now I have to learn to do the checkbook."*

*A husband said, "I feel like a fool washing ladies' under-wear in the laundromat."*

*A son said, "My father has always been the head of the household. How can I tell him he can't drive?"*

*A daughter said, "Why can't my brother help out and take his turn keeping Mother?"*

Roles are different from responsibilities, and it is helpful to recognize what roles mean to you and to others in the family. Responsibilities are the jobs each person has in the family. Roles include who you are, how you are seen, and what is expected of you. By "role" we mean a person's place in his family (e.g., head of the household, mother, or "the person everyone turns to"). Roles are established over many years and are not always easy to define. Tasks often symbolize our roles. In the examples above, family members describe both having to learn new tasks (doing the wash or balancing the checkbook) and changing in roles (money manager, homemaker, head of the household).

Learning a new responsibility, such as keeping the check-book or washing clothes, can be difficult when you are also faced with the many day-to-day needs of the confused person, yourself, and your family. However, changes in roles are often more difficult to accept or adjust to. Understanding that each person's responsibilities change and that roles and expecta-tions of others change also will help you to understand other personal feelings and problems that may arise in families. It is helpful to remember that you have coped with changes in roles at other times in your life and that this experience will help you adjust to new responsibilities.

There are many relationships in which role changes occur as the person becomes demented. Here are four examples.

1. *The relationships between a husband and wife change*

*when one of them becomes ill.* These changes may be sad and painful. Others can be enriching experiences.

*John and Mary Douglas had been married forty-one years when John got sick. John had always been the head of the household: he supported the family, paid the bills, made most of the big decisions. Mary saw herself as a person who always leaned on her husband. When he got sick, she realized that she did not know how much money they had, what insurance they had, or even how to balance a checkbook. Bills were going unpaid, yet when she asked John about it, he yelled at her.*

*For their anniversary Mary fixed a small turkey and planned a quiet time together when they could forget what was happening. When she put the electric carving knife in front of John he threw it down and shouted at her that the knife did not work and she had ruined the turkey. Trying to keep the peace, Mary took the knife, and then realized that she had no idea how to carve a turkey. Mary cried and John stormed. Neither of them felt like eating supper that night.*

Having to carve a turkey seemed like the last straw for Mary. She realized that John could no longer do this, nor could he manage their finances, but she suddenly felt overwhelmed and lost. Throughout their marriage Mary had looked to John to solve problems. Now she had to learn to do the things he had always done at the same time that she had to face his illness.

Learning new skills and responsibilities involves energy and effort and means work added to what you already have to do. You may not want to take on new tasks. Few husbands want to learn to do the wash, and more than one has had a load of shrunken sweaters and pale pink jockey shorts before he finds out that he can't wash red sweaters with white underwear. A spouse who has never managed the checkbook may feel that he doesn't have the ability to manage money and may be afraid of making errors.

In addition to having to do the job itself, the realization that you must take this job away from your spouse may symbolize all of the sad changes that have taken place. For Mary, carving the turkey symbolized John's loss of status as head of the family.

A spouse may gradually realize that he is alone with his problem—he has lost the partner with whom he shared things. Mary could no longer see herself as leaning on her husband. She suddenly found herself, at sixty, on her own and forced to be independent with no one to help her. No wonder she felt overwhelmed by the task. But at the same time, learning new skills gradually gave Mary a sense of accomplishment. She said, "I was surprised at myself, really, that I could handle things. Even though I felt so upset, it was good for me to learn that I could manage so well."

Sometimes problems that seem insurmountable seem that way because they involve both changes in roles and the need for you to learn new tasks. Having to learn new skills when you are upset and tired can be difficult. As well as recognizing the distress that may be caused by changing roles, you may need some practical suggestions for getting started with new responsibilities.

If you must take over the housework, often you can do it gradually and learn as you go. But you can save yourself the frustration of burned suppers and ruined laundry by getting the advice of experts. The county extension office usually has excellent information on shopping, meal preparation, laundry, budgeting, and home maintenance, or you can get advice from homemakers or a visiting nurse. You may even find useful brochures or recipes in the supermarket.

*Mrs. Stearns says, "I know my husband can't manage his money any more, but it seems like it is taking away the last of his manhood to take away the checkbook. I know I have to, but I just can't seem to do it."*

Having to take this symbol of independence away from someone you love can be difficult. It can be worse when you are not accustomed to managing money.

If you have never balanced a checkbook or paid the bills, you may find it hard to learn this new responsibility. Actually, managing household finances is not difficult, even for people who dislike math. Most banks have staff who will advise you, without charge. They also will show you how to balance a checkbook. There are books in the library on this subject. The fact that you must take over this role, rather than the task itself, sometimes is what makes it hard to do.

The bank or a lawyer can also help you draw up a list of yours or the confused person's assets and debts. Sometimes a person has been private about financial affairs, has told no one, and now cannot remember them. Chapter 15 lists some of the potential resources you should look for.

If you can't drive or do not like to drive and must take over the driving responsibilities, look for a driver education course designed for adults. Inquire through the police or the American Association of Retired Persons for driver's education courses and defensive driving programs for older adults. Life will be much easier if you are comfortable behind the wheel.

2. *The relationship of a parent with a dementing illness and his adult children often has to change.* The changes that occur when an adult child must assume the responsibility and care of a parent are sometimes called "role reversal." Perhaps this is better described as a shift in roles and responsibilities, in which the adult son or daughter gradually assumes increasing responsibility for a parent while the roles of the parent change accordingly. These changes can be difficult. You, the adult son or daughter, may feel sadness and grief at the losses you

see in someone you love and look up to. You may feel guilty about "taking over."

*"I can't tell my mother she shouldn't live alone any more,"* Mrs. Russo says. *"I know I have to, but every time I try to talk to her she manages to make me feel like a small child who has been bad."*

To varying degrees many of us as adults still feel that our parents are parents and that we, the children, are less assured, capable, and "grown up." In some families the parents seem to maintain this kind of relationship with their adult children past the time when adult sons and daughters usually come to feel mature in their own right.

Not everyone has had a good relationship with his parents. If a parent has not been able to let his grown children feel grown up, a lot of unhappiness and conflict may develop. Then as the parent develops a dementing illness he can seem to be demanding and manipulative of you. You may find yourself feeling trapped. You may feel used, angry, and guilty at the same time.

What seems demanding to you may feel different to the impaired person. He may be feeling that with "just a little help" he can hold on to his independence, perhaps continue to live alone. As he senses his decline, this may seem the only way he can respond to his losses.

Adult children often feel embarrassed by the tasks of physically caring for a parent—for example, giving their mother a bath or changing their father's underwear. Look for ways to help your parent retain his dignity at the same time that you give needed care.

3. *The sick person must adjust to his changing roles in the family.* This often means giving up some of his independence, responsibility, or leadership, which can be difficult for everyone. (Also see Chapter 4.) He may become discouraged or depressed as he realizes his abilities are waning.

The roles a person has held within the family in the past, and the kind of person he is, will influence the new roles he assumes as he becomes ill. You can help him to maintain his position as an important member of the family even when he can no longer do the tasks he once did. Consult him, talk to him, listen to him (even if what he says seems confused). Let him know by these actions that he is still respected.

4. *As the roles of the sick person change, the expectations of each member of the family for the others change.* Your relationships and expectations of members of the family are based on family roles that have been established for years. Changes often lead to conflicts, misunderstandings, and times when people's expectations of each other do not agree. At the same time, adjusting to changes and facing problems can bring families closer together, even when they have not been close for years.

## UNDERSTANDING FAMILY CONFLICTS

*Mrs. Eaton says, "My brother doesn't have anything to do with Mom now—and he was always her favorite. He won't even come to see her. All the burden is on my sister and me. Because my sister's marriage is shaky, I hate to leave Mom with her for long. So I end up taking care of Mom pretty much alone."*

*Mr. Cooke says, "My son wants me to put her in a nursing home. He doesn't understand that, after thirty years of marriage, I can't just put her in a nursing home." His son says, "Dad isn't being realistic. He can't manage Mother in that big two-story house. She's going to fall one of these days. And Dad has a heart condition that he refuses to discuss."*

*Mr. Vane says, "My brother says if I keep her more active, she would get better. He says I should answer her back when she gets nasty, but that only makes things worse. He*

211

*doesn't live with her. He just stays in his own apartment and criticizes."*

## Division of Responsibility

The responsibility of caring for an impaired person often is not evenly shared by the family. Like Mrs. Eaton, you may find that you are carrying most of the burden of taking care of the person who has a dementing illness. There are many reasons why it is difficult to divide responsibility evenly. Some members of the family may live far away, may be in poor health, may be financially unable to help, or may have problems with their children or marriage.

Sometimes families accept stereotypes about who should help without really considering what is best. One such stereotype is that daughters (and daughters-in-law) are "supposed" to take care of the sick. But the daughter or daughter-in-law may already be heavily burdened and not be able to take on this task. Perhaps she has young children, or a full-time job. Perhaps she is a single parent.

Long-established roles, responsibilities, and mutual expectations within the family, even when we are unaware of them, can play an important part in determining who has what responsibility for the impaired person. For example.

*"My mother raised me; now I must take care of her."*

*"She was a good wife, and she would have done the same for me."*

*"I married him late in life. What responsibility is mine and what responsibility is his children's?"*

*"He was always hard on me, deserted my mother when I was ten, and he's willed all his money to some organization. How much do I owe him?"*

Sometimes expectations are not logical and may not be based on the most practical or fair way to arrange things.

Sometimes family members fail to help as much as they might because it is difficult for them to accept the reality of the impaired person's illness. Sometimes a person just can't bear to face this illness. It is painful, as you know, to watch a loved one decline. Sometimes family members who do not have the burden of daily care stay away because seeing the decline makes them feel sad. However, others in the family may view this as deserting the declining person.

Sometimes one family member assumes most of the burden of care. He may not tell other members of the family how bad things are. He may not want to burden them or he may not really want their help.

*Mr. Newman says, "I hesitate to call on my sons. They are willing to help, but they have their own careers and families."*

*Mrs. King says, "I don't like to call on my daughter. She always tells me what she thinks I am doing wrong."*

Often you and other members of the family have strong and differing ideas of how things should be done. Sometimes this happens because not all family members understand what is wrong with the person who has a dementing illness, or why he acts as he does, or what can be expected in the future.

Family members who do not share the day-to-day experience of living with a person suffering from a dementing illness may not know what it is really like, and may be critical or unsympathetic. It is hard for people on the outside to realize how wearing the daily burden of constant care can be. Often, too, people don't realize how you are feeling unless you tell them.

Sometimes there have been long-established disagreements, resentments, or conflicts in the family which are aggravated by the crisis of an illness.

213

## YOUR MARRIAGE

When the ill person is your parent or in-law, it is important to consider the effect of his illness on your marriage. Maintaining a good marriage is often not easy, and caring for a person with a dementing illness can make it much more difficult. It may mean more financial burdens and less time to talk, to go out, and to make love. It may entail being involved with your in-laws, having more things to disagree over, often being tired, and short-changing the children. It can mean having to include a difficult, disagreeable, seemingly demanding, and sick person in your lives.

A dementing illness can be painful to watch. It is understandable that a person may look at his impaired in-law and wonder if his spouse will become like that, and if he will have to go through this again.

A son or daughter can easily find himself or herself torn between the needs of an impaired parent, the expectations of brothers and sisters (or the other parent), and the needs and demands of a spouse and children. It's easy to take out frustrations or fatigue on those we love and trust most—our spouse and our children.

The spouse of an ill parent may also add problems. He or she may be upset, critical, or ill, or he may even desert his ill partner. Such problems can add to the tension in your marriage, and, if at all possible, should be discussed with everyone involved. It is sometimes easier if a son initiates a solution with his own family or a daughter with her own relatives.

A good relationship can survive for a while in the face of stress and trouble, but we believe it is important that the husband and wife find time and energy for each other—to talk, to get away, and to enjoy their relationship in the ways that they always have.

## COPING WITH ROLE CHANGES AND FAMILY CONFLICT

When the family does not agree, or when most of the burden is on one person, it adds to the problems you face. The burden of caring for a chronically ill person is often too much for one individual. It is important that you have others to help—to give you "time out" from constant care, to give you encouragement and support, to help with the work, and to share the financial responsibility.

If you are getting criticism or not enough help from your family, it is usually not a good idea to let your resentment smolder. It may be up to you to take the initiative to change things in your family. When families are in disagreement or when long-established conflicts get in the way, this may be difficult to do.

How do you handle the often complex, painful role changes that are set in motion by a chronic, dementing illness? First, recognize these as aspects of family relationships. Just knowing that roles in families are complex, often unrecognized or unacknowledged, and that changes can be painful will help you to feel less panicked and overwhelmed. Recognize that certain tasks may be symbolic of important roles in the family and that it is the shift of role, rather than the specific issue, which may be painful.

Find out all you can about the disease. What family members believe to be true about this illness affects how much help they provide for a person and affects whether there will be disagreements about caring for the impaired person.

Think about the differences between the responsibilities or tasks that an impaired person may have to give up and the roles that he may be able to retain. For example, although John's illness means he can no longer carve a turkey or make many decisions, his *role* as Mary's loved and respected husband can remain.

215

Know what the impaired person is still able to do and what is too difficult for him. Of course, one wants a person to remain as self-reliant as possible, but expectations that exceed his abilities can make him upset and miserable. (Sometimes such expectations of how well he can function come from others, sometimes they come from the impaired person himself.) If he cannot do a task independently, try to simplify the job so that he can still do part of it.

Recognize that role changes are not one-time things, but are on-going processes. As the illness progresses, you may continue to have to take on new responsibilities. Each time you will probably reexperience some of the feelings of sadness and of being overwhelmed by your job. This is a part of the grief process in a chronic disease.

Talk over your situation with other families. This is one of the advantages of family support groups. You may find it comforting to learn that other families have struggled with similar changes. Laugh at yourself a little. When you have just burned supper or hacked up a turkey, try to see the humor in the situation. Often where families of people with dementing illnesses get together they share both tears and laughter over such experiences.

Look for ways to help each other. When a wife has most of the responsibility of daily care for an impaired person, she may badly need her husband's help with such untraditional jobs as the housework or sitting with the parent while she goes out. She will certainly need his love and encouragement and may need his help with the rest of the family.

You may reach a point where the extent and demands of your job are exhausting you. You need to be able to recognize this and to make other arrangements when that time comes. Your responsibilities as decision maker may eventually include making the decision to give up your role as primary care giver.

## A Family Conference

We feel that a family conference is one of the most effective ways to help families cope. Have a family meeting, with help from a counselor or the physician if needed, to talk over the problems and to make plans. Together you can make definite decisions about how much help or money each person will contribute.

There are ground rules for a family conference which you might suggest at the beginning: everyone comes (including children who will be affected by the decision), each person has his say uninterrupted, and everyone listens to what the others have to say (even if they don't agree).

If family members disagree about what is wrong with the confused, forgetful person or about how to manage his care, it may be helpful to give other members of the family this book and other written materials about the specific disease, or to ask the doctor to talk with them. It is surprising how often this reduces the tensions between family members.

Here are some questions to ask of each other when you get together. What are the problems? Who is doing what now? What needs to be done, and who can do it? How can you help each other? What will these changes mean for each of you? Some of the practical questions that may need to be discussed might be: Who will be responsible for daily care? Does this mean giving up privacy? not having friends over? not being able to afford a vacation? Does this mean that parents will be busy with the sick person? Who will make the decision to put a parent in a nursing home? Who will be responsible for the sick person's money?

If a well spouse of the impaired person is to move into a son or daughter's home with the impaired person, what will this person's roles in the family be? Will she have responsibility for the grandchildren? Will there be two women in the kitchen? An expanded family can be enriching but it also can create tensions. Anticipating and discussing areas of disagreement in advance can make things easier.

It is also important to talk about several other practical areas in which family relationships can get into trouble. It can seem insensitive even to think about matters of money or inheritance when a loved one is sick. But financial concerns are important, and questions about who will get the inheritance are real—if often hidden—factors in determining responsibility for a family member. They can be the underlying cause of much bitterness. Money matters need to be brought out in the open. Ask yourself the following questions.

Does everyone know what money and inheritance there is? It is surprising how often one son is thinking, "Dad has that stock he bought twenty years ago, he owns his house, and he has his social security. He ought to be quite comfortable." The other son, who is taking care of his father, knows "the house needs a new roof and a new furnace, that old mining stock is worthless, and he gets barely enough to live on from social security. I have to dip into my own pocket to pay for his medicine."

Is there a will? Does someone know or suspect that he has been shortchanged in the will? Do some members of the family feel that others are greedy for inherited money, property, or personal possessions? This is not unusual and it can best be handled when it is openly faced. Hidden resentments often smolder and can emerge as conflicts over the daily care of the person.

How much does it cost to care for the sick person and who is paying these bills? When a family cares for a person at home, there are many "hidden" costs to consider; special foods, medication, special door latches, a sitter, transportation, another bed and a dresser on the ground floor, grab bars for the bathroom, perhaps the cost of a wife's not working because she must care for the confused person.

Does everyone know what it costs to care for a person with a dementing illness in a nursing home, and does everyone know who is legally responsible for those costs? (We have discussed nursing home costs in Chapter 16.) Sometimes when a daughter says, "Mother must put Dad in a nursing home," she does not realize that doing so may deprive her mother of most of their joint income and leave her mother nearly destitute.

Do some members of the family feel that money has been unequally distributed in the past? For example.

*"Dad put my brother through college and gave him the down payment on his house. Yet now my brother won't take him, so I get the work—and the cost—of taking care of him."*

Families sometimes say, "There is no way you'll get my family together to talk about things like that. My brother won't even discuss it on the phone. And if we did get together it could just be a big fight." If you feel that your family is like this, you may be discouraged. Although you need your family's help, you may feel trapped because you feel that your family will not help. It is not unusual for families to need the help of an outside person—a counselor, minister, or social worker—to help work out their problems and to help them arrive at equitable arrangements. (See p. 261.)

One of the advantages of seeking the assistance of a counselor is that he can listen objectively and help the family to keep the discussion on the problems you face and not drift aside into old arguments. Your doctor, a social worker, or a counselor may be able to intervene on your behalf and convince everyone involved of the need for a family to discuss issues of concern to them all. Sometimes a family attorney can help. If you seek the help of an attorney, be sure that he is genuinely interested in helping resolve conflict rather than helping you get into litigation against your own family. If a family is having difficulty and you ask a third party to help you, the first topic of conversation may be to agree that the third party will not take sides with any one person.

You need your family. Now is an excellent time to put aside old conflicts for the sake of the impaired person. Perhaps if your family cannot resolve all your disagreements, you can, in a discussion, find one or two things upon which you agree. This will encourage everyone and the next discussion may be easier.

## YOUR CHILDREN

Having children at home can create special problems. They, too, have a relationship with the sick person, and they have complex feelings—which they may not express—about his illness and roles in the family. Parents often worry about the effect that being around a person with a dementing illness will have on children. It is hard to know what to tell a child about a parent's or grandparent's "odd" behavior. Sometimes parents worry that children will learn undesirable behavior from people with dementing illnesses.

Children are usually aware of what is going on. They are excellent observers and, even when things are carefully concealed from them, often sense that something is wrong. Fortunately, children are marvelously resilient. Even small children can benefit from an honest explanation of what is happening to the person with a dementing illness—in language they can understand. This helps them not to be frightened. Reassure the child that this illness is not "catching" like chickenpox and that neither the children nor his parents are likely to get it. Tell the child directly that nothing he did "caused" this illness. Sometimes children secretly feel to blame for the things that happen in their family.

*One father put a pile of dried beans on the table. He took little pieces of the pile away as he gave his young son the following explanation of his grandfather's illness: "Grandpop has a sickness that makes him act like he does. It isn't catching. None of us is going to get like Grandpop. It's like having a broken leg, only little pieces of Grandpop's brain are broken. He won't get any better. This little piece of Grandpop's brain is broken, so he can't remember what you just told him; this little piece is broken, so he forgets how to use his silverware at the table; this little piece is broken, so he gets mad real easy. But this part, which is for loving, Grandpop still has left."*

It is usually best to involve children actively in what is happening in the family and even to find ways in which they can help. Small children frequently relate well to impaired, confused people, and can establish special and loving relationships with them. Try to create an atmosphere in which the child can ask you questions and express his feelings openly. Remember that children also feel sadness and grief, but they may be able to enjoy the childlike ways of an impaired person without feeling at all sad. The more comfortable you feel in your understanding of this illness, the more easily you will be able to explain it to your child.

Children may need help knowing what to tell playmates who tease them about a "funny" parent or grandparent.

It is unlikely that children will mimic the undesirable behaviors of a person with a dementing illness for long if you don't make a big deal out of this if it happens and if the child is getting enough love and attention. Clearly explain (probably several times) to the child that his parent or grandparent has a disease and cannot help what he does but that the child can, and is expected to, control his behavior.

Young people may be frightened by unexplained, strange behavior. Sometimes they worry that something they did or might do will make the person worse. If is important to talk about these concerns and to reassure the young person.

One family with children ranging from ten to sixteen shared with us the following thoughts based on their own experience:

What's going on in a child's head is not what we think! Anyone who has been around children much can think of examples of this. Don't assume that you know what a youngster is thinking.

Children, even small children, also feel pity, sadness, and sympathy.

If we had it to do over again, we would talk more with the children.

The effects of this illness linger long after the confused person has gone to a nursing home. Get together with the children afterward and continue to discuss things.

Make an effort to involve all of the children equally in the person's care. Children can find it hard to be depended on or they can feel left out. Sharing in care gives them a sense of responsibility.

The parent closest to the sick person needs to be aware of the children and the effect of her grief and distress on them. Sometimes a person can be so overwhelmed by her own troubles that she forgets the children. Her behavior can be as hard on the children as the illness itself.

Perhaps the biggest problem when there are children at home is that the parent's time and energies are divided between that person and the children—with never enough for both. In order to cope with this double load you will need every bit of help available—the help of the rest of the family, the resources of the community, and time—for you to replenish your own emotional and physical energies. You may find yourself torn between neglecting the children and neglecting a "childish" or demanding person with a dementing illness.

As the person's condition worsens, so may your dilemma. The declining person may need more and more care, and may be so disruptive that chldren cannot feel comfortable at home. You may not have the physical or emotional energy to meet the needs of children or adolescents and the sick person. Children growing up in such a situation may suffer as a result of the person's illness.

You may make the painful decision to place the sick person in a nursing home in order to create a better home environment for the children. If you face such a decision, you and your children need to discuss what is to be done, talking over what your alternatives will mean to each member of the family. "We will have less money for movies, but we wouldn't have Dad shouting all night." "We would move and have to change schools, but I could bring friends home."

The support of your doctor, clergy, or a counselor is helpful at such times. Families often find it easier to make decisions when they know they are not alone.

## Teenagers

Adolescents may be embarrassed by "odd" behavior, reluctant to bring friends home, resentful of the demands made on you by the confused person, or hurt by the confused person's failure to remember them. Adolescents can also be extraordinarily compassionate, supportive, responsible, and altruistic. They often have an unspoiled sense of humanitarianism and kindness which is refreshing and helpful. Certainly they will have mixed feelings. Like you, they may experience the grief of seeing someone they love change drastically at the same time that they may feel resentful or embarrassed. Mixed feelings lead to mixed actions that are often puzzling to other family members. Adolescent years can be hard for young people, whether there are problems at home or not. However, many adults, looking back, recognize that sharing in family problems helped them to become mature adults.

Be sure your adolescent understands the nature of the disease and what is happening. Be honest with him about what is going on. Explanations, given gently, help a lot. Children seldom benefit from mistaken attempts to shelter them. Involve the adolescent in the family discussions, groups, and conferences with health professionals, so that he, too, understands what is happening.

Take time away from the sick person, when you are not exhausted or cross, to maintain a good relationship with your adolescent and to listen to his interests. Remember that he has a life apart from this illness and this situation. Try to find space for his teenage friends apart from the impaired person.

Remember that you may be less patient or more emotional because of all you are dealing with. Again, breaks for you may help you be more patient with your children.

When a grandparent moves into your home, it is important that both he and your children know who sets the rules and who disciplines the children. When the grandparent is forgetful, it is important that your children know *from you* what is expected of them to avoid conflicts like, "Grandmother says I can't date." "Granddad says I have to turn off the TV."

# 12

## How Caring For An Impaired Person Affects You

FAMILY MEMBERS TELL US that they experience many feelings as they care for a person with a chronic, dementing illness. They feel sad, discouraged, and alone. They feel angry, guilty, or hopeful. They feel tired or depressed. In the face of the reality of a chronic illness, emotional distress is appropriate and understandable. Sometimes families of people with dementing illnesses find themselves overwhelmed by their feelings.

Human feelings are complex and they vary with each person. In this chapter we have tried to avoid oversimplifying feelings or offering simplistic solutions. Our goal is to remind you that it is not unusual to experience many feelings.

### EMOTIONAL REACTIONS

People have different ways of handling their emotions. Some people experience each feeling intensely; others do not.

Sometimes people think that certain feelings are unacceptable—that they should not have certain feelings or that, if they do, no one could possibly understand them. Sometimes they feel alone with their feelings.

Sometimes people have mixed feelings. One might both love and dislike the same person, or want to keep a family member at home and put her in a nursing home, all at the same time. Having mixed feelings might not seem logical but it is common. Often people do not realize that they have mixed feelings.

Sometimes people are afraid of strong emotions, perhaps because such feelings are uncomfortable, perhaps because they are afraid they might do something rash, or perhaps because they are concerned about how others will view them. These and other responses to our feelings are not unusual. In fact, most of us will have similar responses at one time or another.

We do not believe there is a "right" way to handle emotions. We think that recognizing how you feel and having some understanding of why you feel the way you do are important, because your feelings affect your judgment. Unrecognized or unacknowledged feelings can influence the decisions a person makes in ways that he does not understand or recognize. You can acknowledge and recognize your feelings—to yourself and to others—but you have a choice of when, where, and whether to express your feelings or to act on them.

People sometimes worry that not expressing feelings causes "stress-related" diseases. Suppose you know that you are often angry with the behavior of a person with a dementing illness, but you decide not to yell at her because it only makes her behavior worse. Will you develop ulcers, or migraines, or hypertension? Researchers disagree about the relationship between expressing feelings and diseases. However, at present, the causes of diseases such as ulcers, migraines, and hypertension are unknown. It has not been our observation that these conditions are more common among families who care for people with dementing illnesses. We do believe that as families recognize that the irritating behaviors of a confused person are symptoms of her disease, they feel less frustrated and angry and they can care better for the confused person.

As you read this section, remember that each person and each family is different. You may not have these feelings. We have discussed them in order to help those family members who do feel angry or discouraged, tired or sad, etc. Rather than read all this material, you may want to refer to it when you feel a particular section will help you.

## Anger

It is understandable that you feel frustrated and angry: angry that this has happened to you, angry that you have to be the care giver, angry with others who don't seem to be helping out, angry with the sick person for her irritating behavior, angry that you are trapped in this situation.

Some people with dementing illness develop behaviors that are extremely irritating and that can seem impossible to live with. You will understandably get angry and may sometimes react by yelling or arguing.

*Mrs. Palombo felt that she must not get angry with her husband. They had had a good marriage and she knew that he could not help himself now that he was ill. She says, "We went to dinner at my daughter-in-law's house. I have never felt comfortable with my daughter-in-law, anyway, and I don't think she understands about Joe. As soon as we got in the door Joe looked around and said, 'Let's go home.' I tried to explain to him that we were staying for dinner and all he would say is, 'I've never liked it here. Let's go home.'*

227

*"We sat down to dinner and everyone was tense. Joe wouldn't talk to anyone and he wouldn't take his hat off. As soon as dinner was over he wanted to go home. My daughter-in-law went in the kitchen and shut the door and started banging the dishes. My son made me go in the den with him and all the time Joe was hollering, 'Let's get out of here before she poisons us.'*

*"My son says I'm letting Dad ruin my life, that there is no reason for Dad to act that way, that that isn't sickness, it's that he's gotten spiteful in his old age. He says I have to do something.*

*"So we got in the car to go home and all the way home Joe hollered at me about my driving, which he always does. As soon as we got home he started asking me what time it was. I said, 'Joe, please be quiet. Go watch television.' And he said, 'Why don't you ever talk to me?' Then I started yelling at him and I yelled and yelled."*

Episodes like this can wear out even the most patient person. It seems as if they always start when we are most tired.

The things that are most irritating sometimes seem like little things—but little things mount up, day after day.

*Mrs. Jackson tells, "I had never gotten along with my mother that well, and since she's come to live with us, it's been terrible. In the middle of the night she gets up and starts packing.*

*"I get up and tell her, 'It's the middle of the night, Mother,' and I try to explain to her that she lives here now, but I'm thinking if I don't get my sleep I won't be any good at work tomorrow.*

*"She says she has to go home, and I say she lives here, and every night a fight starts at two o'clock in the morning."*

Sometimes a person with a dementing illness can do some things very well and appear unwilling to do other, seemingly identical tasks. When you feel that the sick person can do more or is just acting up to "get your goat," it can be infuriating. For example,

*Mrs. Graham says, "She can load the dishwasher and set the table just fine at my sister's house but at my house she either refuses to do it or she makes a terrible mess. Now I know it's because I work and she knows I come home tired."*

Often the person who has most of the responsibility for the care of a sick person feels that other members of the family don't help out enough, are critical, or don't come to visit. A lot of anger can build up around these feelings.

You may be irritated with doctors and other professionals at times. Sometimes your anger toward them is legitimate; at other times you may know that they are doing the best they can, yet you are still angry with them.

People with a religious faith may question how God could allow this to happen to them. They may feel that it is a terrible sin to be angry with God or they may fear that they have lost their faith. Such feelings may deprive them of the strength and reassurance faith offers at just the time when they need it most. To struggle with such questions is part of the experience of faith.

*Said a minister, "I wonder how God could do this to me. I haven't been perfect; but I've done the best I could. And I love my wife. But then I think I have no right to question God. For me that is the hardest part. I think I must be a very weak person to question God."*

Never let a person make you feel guilty for your anger with God. There are many thoughtful and meaningful writings discussing such things as feeling anger with God or questioning how He could do such a thing as this. C. S. Lewis's book *A Grief Observed* eloquently describes his own struggle with these questions. Reading this and other books, and talking honestly with your minister, priest, or rabbi can be comforting.

Remember, it is only human to be angry when faced with the burdens and losses a dementing illness often brings.

Expressing your anger to the sick person often makes her behavior worse. Her illness may make it impossible for her to respond to your anger in a rational way. You may find that it improves her behavior when you find other ways to manage both your frustrations and the problems themselves.

The first step in dealing with anger is to know what you can reasonably expect from a person with a dementing illness, and what is happening to the brain to cause irritating behavior. If you are not sure whether the person can stop acting the way she does, find out from your doctor or other professional staff. For example,

*An occupational therapist discovered that Mrs. Graham's sister had an old dishwasher that her mother had operated before she got sick. Mrs. Graham had a new dishwasher that her mother could not learn to use because her brain impairment made it impossible for her to learn even simple new skills.*

It may be possible to change the person's irritating behavior by changing the environment or the daily routine. However, just knowing that unpleasant behavior is the result of the disease that the person cannot help can be reassuring.

It is often helpful to think about the difference between being angry with the person's *behavior* and being angry with the *person herself*. She is ill and often cannot stop her behavior. Certainly, the behavior can be infuriating, but it is not aimed at you personally.

A dementing illness might make it impossible for a person to be deliberately offensive because she has lost the ability to take purposeful action. Mrs. Palombo's husband was not deliberately insulting his family. His behavior was the result of his illness.

It often helps to know that other families and professional care givers have the same problems.

*Says Mrs. Kurtz, "I didn't want to put my husband in day care, but I did it. It helped me so much to find out that his constant questions made trained professionals angry too. It wasn't just me."*

Many families find that discussing their experiences with other families helps them to feel less frustrated and upset.

Sometimes it is helpful to find other outlets for your frustrations: talking to someone about it, cleaning closets, or chopping wood—whatever ways you have used in the past to cope with your frustrations. A vigorous exercise program, a long walk, or taking a few minutes to relax totally may be helpful for you.

## Helplessness

It is not uncommon for family members to feel helpless, weak, or demoralized in the face of a chronic dementing illness. These feelings are often made worse when you cannot find doctors or other professionals who seem to understand dementing illnesses. We have found that families and the people with dementing illnesses have many resources within themselves with which they can overcome feelings of helplessness. Although you may not be able to cure the disease, you are far from helpless. There are many ways to improve life for both the forgetful person and the family. Here are some places to start.

Things often seem worse when you look at everything at once. Instead, focus on changing small things that you can change.

Take one day at a time.

Be informed about the disease. Read and talk about ways others manage.

Talk with other families who face similar problems.

Get involved in exchanging information, supporting research, and reaching others.

Discuss your feelings with the doctor, social worker, psychologist, or clergyman.

## Embarrassment

Sometimes the behavior of a person with a dementing illness is embarrassing and strangers often do not understand what is happening.

*Says Mrs. McGregor, "I say my husband has Alzheimer's disease. 'Old timer's disease?' they say. 'No, Alzheimer's disease!' I say, and I spell it. If my husband had a brain tumor they would understand. How I wish he didn't have a disease nobody ever heard of!"*

*Says one husband, "Going through the grocery store, she keeps taking things down off the shelves like a toddler, and people stare."*

*Says a daughter, "Every time we try to give Mother a bath she opens the window and shouts for help. What are we to tell the neighbors?"*

Such experiences *are* embarrassing, although much of your embarrassment may fade as you share your experiences with other families. In such groups families often find they laugh over things like this.

Explaining to neighbors usually helps gain their understanding. You might give them copies of the "handouts" about these diseases. There is another reason why this is important. Although these dementing diseases are common, many people still think "senility" is the natural result of getting older. By explaining the illness to your neighbors you are helping get these diseases out of the closet. Your neighbor may well know someone else with one of these diseases who needs treatment.

Occasionally, some insensitive person will ask a rude question, such as "Why does he act like that?" or "Whatever is wrong with her?" Sometimes it may be most effective to say "Whyever would you ask?"

*One courageous husband says, "I still take my wife out to dinner. I don't like to cook and she likes to go out. I ignore other people's glances. This is something we always enjoyed doing together, and we still do!"*

## Guilt

It is quite common for family members to feel guilty: for the way they treated the person in the past; for being embarrassed by the person's "odd" behavior; for losing their temper with a sick person; for not wanting this responsibility; for considering placing the person in a nursing home; and for many other reasons, some trivial, some enormous. For example.

*"My mother's illness ruined my marriage and I can't forgive her for it."*

You may feel guilty about your occasional angry outbursts when you are frustrated with the impaired person.

*"I lost my temper with Dick and slapped him. Yet I know he is sick and can't help himself."*

You may feel guilty about spending time with your friends away from the person you love, especially when the person is your spouse and you have been accustomed to doing most things together.

You may feel vaguely guilty without knowing why. Sometimes people feel that the person with a dementing illness *makes* them feel guilty. "Promise me that you will never put me in a nursing home," or "You wouldn't treat me that way if you loved me" is something the confused person may say that can make you feel guilty.

Sometimes we feel guilty when a person close to us, whom we have always disliked, develops a dementing disease:

*"I've never liked my mother and now she has this terrible disease. If only I had been closer to her when I could."*

Families sometimes ask if something they did or failed to do caused the illness. Sometimes the caretaking person feels responsible when the person gets worse. You may feel that if only you had taken more time with her or kept her more active she would not have gotten worse. You may feel that surgery or a hospitalization "caused" this condition.

The trouble with feelings of guilt is that, when they are not recognized for what they are, they can keep you from making clear-headed decisions about the future and doing what is right for the sick person and the rest of the family. When such feelings are recognized, they are not surprising or hard to manage.

The first step is to admit that feelings of guilt *are* a problem. They become a problem when they affect your decisions. If you are being influenced by guilt feelings, you must make a decision. Are you going to go around in a circle with one foot caught in the trap of guilt, or are you going to say "What is done is done" and go on from there? Often, the fact that you never liked your mother or that you slapped a sick person, for example. However, guilt feelings tend to keep us looking for ways to remedy the past instead of letting us accept the fact that you can stop trying to make up for your guilt feelings and instead make decisions and plans based on what is best now. For example.

*Mrs. Dempsey had never liked her mother. As soon as she could she had moved away from home and called her mother only on special occasions. When her mother developed a dementing illness, she brought her mother to live with her. The confused woman disrupted the family, kept everyone up at night, upset the children, and left Mrs. Dempsey exhausted. When the doctor recommended that her mother enter a nursing home, Mrs. Dempsey only became more upset. She could not bring herself to put her mother in a nursing home even though this clearly would be better for everyone.*

When the feelings of guilt in such a relationship are not acknowledged, they can destructively affect how you act. Perhaps being faced with a chronic illness is a good time to be honest with yourself about not liking someone. You can then choose whether to give a person care and respect without being influenced by not liking her. We have little control over whom we like or love. Some people are not very likeable, but we do have control over how we act toward them. When Mrs. Dempsey was able to face the fact that she did not like her mother and that she felt guilty about that, she was able to go ahead and arrange for her mother to get good nursing home care.

When the person with a dementing illness says things like "Promise you won't put me in a nursing home,' it is helpful to remember that sometimes the person with a dementing illness *cannot* make responsible decisions and that you must make the decisions, acting not on the basis of guilt but on the basis of your responsibility.

Not all feelings of guilt are over major issues or keep you from making good decisions. Sometimes you may feel guilty about little things—being cross with the confused person or snapping at her when you are tired. Saying "I'm sorry" often clears the air and makes you both feel better. Often the confused person, because he is forgetful, will have forgotten the incident long before you have.

If you worry that you have caused this illness or made it worse, it is helpful to learn all you can about the disease and to talk over the person's illness with her doctor.

In general, Alzheimer's disease is a progressive illness. Neither you nor your physician can prevent this progression. It may not be possible to stop or reverse a multi-infarct dementia either. Keeping a person active will not stop the progress of such a disease, but it can help the person use her remaining abilities.

A person's condition may first become apparent after an illness or hospitalization, but often, upon close examination, the beginning stages of the illness occurred months or years earlier. At present, earlier identification of Alzheimer's disease does not help to slow or reverse its progression.

If you don't feel right about doing things for yourself and by yourself, remind yourself that it is important for the confused person's well-being that your life have meaning and fulfillment outside of caring for her. Rest and the companionship of friends will do much to keep you going.

When guilt feelings are keeping you from making clearheaded decisions, you may find it helpful to talk the whole thing out with an understanding counselor, a minister, or other families so that you can go on more easily. Learning that most people do similar things helps to put little nagging guilt feelings in their proper perspective.

## Laughter, Love, and Joy

A dementing illness does not suddenly end a person's capacity to experience love or joy, nor does it end her ability to laugh. And although your life may often seem filled with fatigue, frustration, or grief, your capacity for these emotions is not gone either. Happiness may seem out of place in the face of trouble, but in fact it crops up unexpectedly. The words of a song written by Sister Miriam Theresa Winter of the Medical Mission Sisters reflect this:

*I saw raindrops on my window*
*Joy is like the rain*
*Laughter runs across my pain,*
*slips away and comes again.*
*Joy is like the rain.*

Laughter might be called a gift to help our sanity in the face of trouble. There is no reason to feel badly if you laugh about the mistakes a confused person makes. She may share the laughter even if she is not sure what is funny.

Fortunately love is not dependent upon intellectual abilities. Focus on the ways you and others still share expressions of affection with the impaired person.


## Grief

As the person's illness progresses and the person changes, you may experience the loss of a companion and a relationship that was important to you. You may grieve for the "way she used to be." You may find yourself feeling sad or discouraged. Sometimes little things may make you feel sad or can start you crying. You may feel that tearfulness or sadness is welling up inside you. Often such feelings come and go, so that you alternate between feeling sad and feeling hopeful. Feelings of sadness are often mixed with feelings of depression or fatigue. Such feelings are a normal part of grieving.

We usually think of grief as an emotional experience that follows a death. However, grief actually is an emotional response to loss and so is a normal experience for people who love a person with a chronic illness.

Grief associated with a death may be an overwhelming grief in the beginning, and gradually lessen. Grief associated with a chronic illness seems to go on and on. Your feelings may shift back and forth between hope that the person will get better and anger and sadness over an irreversible condition. Just when you think you have "adjusted," the person may change and you will go through the grieving experience over again. Whether it is the grief that follows death or that which comes with being with a person with a dementing illness, grief is a feeling associated with losing those qualities of a person who was important to you.

Families often say that their own sadness at losing a loved one is made worse because they must watch the suffering of the person as her illness progresses.

*Says Mrs. Owens, "Sometimes I wish he would die so it would be over. It seems as if he is dying a bit at a time, day after day. When something new happens I think I can't stand it. Then I get used to it, and something else happens. And I keep hoping—for a new doctor, a new treatment, maybe a miracle. It seems like I'm on an emotional treadmill going around and around and it's slowly wearing me down."*

There are certain changes that come with a chronic dementing illness which seem especially hard to bear. Particular characteristics of the people we love symbolize for us who that person is: "He was always the one who made decisions" or "She was always such a friendly person." When these things change, they may precipitate feelings of sadness which are sometimes not understood by people less close to the situation. For example, when a person is unable to talk or understand clearly, her family may acutely feel the loss of her companionship.

A husband or wife has lost the spouse he or she used to have but is not a single person. This creates a special set of problems, which we will discuss below, in the section "You as a Spouse Alone."

Another problem is that the grief that follows a death is understood and accepted by society, while the grief that comes with a chronic illness is often misunderstood by friends and neighbors, especially when the ill person looks well. Your loss then is not as visible as it is in a death. "Be grateful you still have your husband," or "Keep a stiff upper lip," people may say.

There are no easy antidotes for grief. Perhaps you will find, as others have, that it is eased somewhat when it is shared with other people who are also living with the unique tragedy of a dementing illness. You may feel that you should keep feelings of sadness and grief to yourself and not burden others with your troubles. However, sharing these feelings can be comforting and can give you the strength you need to continue to care for a declining person.

## Depression

Depression is a feeling of sadness and discouragement. It is often difficult to distinguish between depression and grief, or between depression and anger, or depression and worry. Families of the chronically ill often feel sad, depressed, discouraged, or low, day after day, week after week. Sometimes they feel apathetic or listless. Depressed people may also feel anxious, nervous, or irritable. Sometimes they don't have much appetite and have trouble sleeping at night. The experience of being depressed is painful; we feel miserable and wish for relief from our sad feelings.

A chronic dementing illness takes its toll on our emotions and provides a real reason for feeling low. Sometimes counseling helps reduce the depression you experience, but counseling cannot cure the situation that has made you depressed; it can only help you deal with it. Many families find that it helps to share experiences and emotions with other families in support groups. Others find that it helps to get away from the sick person and spend time with hobbies or people they enjoy. When you are unable to get enough rest, your fatigue may make your feelings of discouragement worse. Getting help so that you can rest may cheer you up. Still, the feelings of discouragement and depression may stick with you—understandably.

For a few people depression goes beyond—or is different from—the understandable feelings of discouragement caused by this illness. Then it is important to consult a physician. He can help significantly with this sort of depression. If any or several of the things listed on page 258 are happening to you or to someone else in the family, it is important to find a physician who can help you or who can refer you to a counselor.

## Isolation; Feeling Alone

Sometimes a family member feels that he is facing this alone. "Despair," one wife said to us. "Write about that feeling of being alone with this." You may feel very much alone when the one person with whom you could share things has changed. You may feel that you must face his illness all alone.

This is a miserable feeling. We are all individuals and no one else can truly understand what we are going through. The feeling of being alone is not uncommon when people are facing a dementing illness. Remaining involved with others—your family, your friends, other people with ill relatives—can help you feel less alone. Sharing experiences with them will help you to realize that others have similar feelings of aloneness. While you may feel that you can never replace the relationship you had with the confused person, you will gradually find that friends and family are offering love and support.

## Worry

Who doesn't worry? We could fill many pages with things families worry about, but you already know them. They are real worries, serious concerns. Worry combines with depression and fatigue and is a fact of life for families. Each person has his own way of coping with worries: some people seem to shrug off serious problems, others seem to fret interminably over trivia, most of us fall somewhere in between. Most of us have also discovered that the kind of worrying we do when we lie awake at night does not solve the problem but it does make us tired. Some of this kind of worrying is often inevitable, but if you are doing a lot of it, you may want to take yourself in hand and look for other ways to manage your problems.

*A woman who faces some real and terrible possibilities in her life tries this approach to worry: "I ask myself what is the worst thing that could happen. We could run out of money and lose our home. But I know people wouldn't let us starve or go homeless. It seems like I don't worry as much once I've faced what the worst could be."*

## Being Hopeful and Being Realistic

As you struggle with a dementing disease, you may find yourself sometimes chasing down every possible hope for a cure and other times feeling discouraged and defeated. You may find yourself unable to accept bad news the doctors have given you. Instead, you may seek second, third, and even more medical opinions at great expense to yourself and the sick person. You may find yourself refusing to believe that anything is wrong. You may even find yourself giggling or acting silly when you really don't have anything to laugh about. Such feelings are normal and are usually a part of our mind's efforts to come to terms with something we don't want to have happen.

Sometimes, of course, ignoring the problem can endanger the sick person (for example, if she is driving or living alone when she cannot do so safely). Seeking many medical opinions can be futile, exhausting, and expensive, but sometimes seeking a second opinion may be wise.

This experience of a mixture of hope and discouragement is common to many families. The problem is complicated when professionals give conflicting information about dementing illnesses.

Most families find reasonable peace in a compromise between hope and realism. How do you know what to do?

Know that we may be a long way from a major research breakthrough or we may be close. Miracles do happen, and yet not often.

Ask yourself if you are going from doctor to doctor or if your reaction is making things more difficult or even risky for the confused person. If you are ignoring her impairments, is she endangering herself by driving, cooking, or continuing to live alone?

Put the sick person in the care of a physician whom you trust. Make sure that this physician is knowledgeable about dementing illnesses and keeps himself abreast of current research. Avoid quack "cures."

Keep yourself informed about the progress of legitimate research. Join the Alzheimer's Disease and Related Disorders Association and local groups to keep abreast of new knowledge.

## PHYSICAL REACTIONS

### Fatigue

Fatigue often comes with depression. It is difficult to know which comes first. People who care for a person with a dementing illness are often tired simply because they aren't getting enough rest. However, being tired adds to the feelings of depression. At the same time, being depressed may make you feel more tired. Always feeling tired is a problem for many people who care for a person with a dementing illness.

Do what you can in little ways to help yourself be less exhausted. For example.

*Mrs. Levin says, "He gets up in the night and puts his hat on and sits on the sofa. I used to wear myself out to get him back to bed. Now I just let him sit there. If he wants to wear his hat with his pajamas, it's O.K. I don't worry about it. I used to think I had to do my windows twice a year and my kitchen floor every week. Now I don't. I have to spend my energy on other things."*

It is important to your health that the person sleep at night or at least be safe at night if she is awake. (We discuss this problem in more detail in Chapter 7: "Sleep Disturbances.") If you are regularly up in the night and still caring for the person all day, your body is paying a price in exhaustion, and you will not be able to keep up such a routine indefinitely. We know that you cannot always get enough rest. However, it is important that you recognize your own limits. We have made suggestions throughout this book which will help you find ways to avoid complete exhaustion.

## Illness

Illness is a camp follower of depression and fatigue. It often seems that people who are discouraged and tired are sick more frequently than others. And people who aren't feeling well are more tired and discouraged. When someone else is dependent on you for care, your sickness can become a serious problem. Who takes care of the confused person when you have the flu? You, probably. You may feel that you have no choice but to keep on dragging yourself around and hope you don't wear out.

Our bodies and our minds are not separate entities; neither is one the slave of the other. They are both parts that make up a whole person, and that whole person can be made less vulnerable—but not invulnerable—to disease.

Do what you can to reduce fatigue and get enough rest. Eat a well-balanced diet. Get anough exercise.

Arrange to take a vacation or to have some time away from your duties as care giver.

Avoid abusing yourself with alcohol, drugs, or overeating. Get an expert—a good physician—to check your routinely for hidden problems such as high blood pressure or anemia and chronic low-grade infections.

Few of us do all that we can to maintain good health even when we have no other serious problems. When you are caring for a chronically ill person, there is often not enough time, energy, or money to go around, and it is yourself that you most often cut short. However, for your sake, and, very importantly, for the sick person's sake, you must do what you can to maintain your health.

## SEXUALITY

It can seem insensitive to think about your own sexuality when there are so many pressing worries—a chronic illness, financial concerns, and so forth. However, people have a life-long need to be loved and touched, and sexuality is a part of our adulthood. It deserves to be considered. Sometimes sex becomes a problem in a dementing illness, but sometimes it remains one of the good things a couple still enjoys. This section is for those couples for whom it has become a problem. Do not read this *expecting* a problem to develop.

## If Your Spouse Is Impaired

Despite the so-called sexual revolution, most people, including many physicians, are uncomfortable talking about sex, especially when it involves older people or handicapped people. This embarrassment, combined with misconceptions about human sexuality, can leave the spouse or companion of a person with a dementing illness alone in silence. Many articles on sex are no help; the subject often cannot be discussed with one's friends, and, if one gets up the courage to ask the doctor, he may quickly change the subject.

At the same time, sexual problems, like many other problems, are often easier to face when they can be acknowledged and talked over with an understanding person.

The spouse of a brain-impaired person may find it impossible to enjoy a sexual relationship when so many other aspects of the relationship have changed so drastically. For many people their sexual relationship can only be good when the whole relationship is good. You may be unable to make love with a person with whom you can no longer enjoy sharing conversation, for example. It may not seem "right" to enjoy sex with a person who has changed so much.

When you are feeling overwhelmed by the tasks of caring for a sick person, when you are tired and depressed, you may be totally uninterested in sex. Sometimes the person with the dementing illness is depressed or moody and loses interest in sex. If this happens early, before the correct diagnosis has been made, it can be misinterpreted as trouble in the relationship.

Sometimes the sexual behavior of a person with a brain disorder may change in ways that are hard for his partner to accept or manage. When the impaired person cannot remember things for more than a few minutes, she may still be able to make love, and want to make love, but will almost immediately forget when it is over, leaving her spouse or partner heartbroken and alone. A few such experiences can make you want to end this aspect of life forever.

Sometimes the person you have cared for all day may say "Who are you? What are you doing in my bed?" Such things can be heartbreaking.

Memory loss can sometimes cause a formerly gentle and considerate person to forget the happy preliminaries to sex. This, too, can be discouraging for the partner.

Occasionally a brain injury or brain disease will cause a person to become sexually demanding. It can be devastating to a spouse when a person who needs so much care in other ways makes frequent demands for sex. When the sexual behavior of a person with a dementing illness changes, this very likely relates to the brain injury or brain damage and is something the person cannot help, rather than being a purposeful affront to your relationship.

Often what people miss most is not the act of sexual intercourse but the touching, holding, and affection that exist between two people. Sometimes, for practical reasons, the well spouse chooses to sleep in a separate room. Sometimes a formerly affectionate person will no longer accept affection when he becomes ill.

*Mr. Bishop says, "We always used to touch each other in our sleep. Now if I put my arm across her she jerks away."*

What can you do about problems of sexuality? Like many of the other problems, there are no easy answers.

It is important that you understand from your spouse's physician the nature of her brain damage and how it affects this and all other aspects of behavior. If you seek help with this problem, be sure the counselor is qualified. Since sexuality is such a sensitive issue, some counselors are not comfortable discussing it or they give inappropriate advice. The counselor should have experience addressing the sexual concerns of handicapped people and should be aware of his own feelings about sexual activity in elderly or handicapped people. There are excellent counselors who have talked about sexuality with many families and who will not be shocked or surprised at what you say. There are also some insensitive people posing as sex counselors whom you will want to avoid.

## If Your Impaired Parent Lives with You

So far we have discussed the problems of the spouse of a person with a dementing illness. However, if your ill parent has come to live with you, the sexual aspect of your marriage can be badly disrupted, and this can affect other areas of your relationship. You may be too tired to make love, or you may have stopped going out together in the evening and thus lost the romance that precedes love making. Your confused parent may wander around the house at night, banging things, knocking on your door, or shouting. The least little noise may rouse the parent you tried so hard to get to sleep. Love making can turn into hurried sex when you are too tired to care, or it can cease altogether.

Relationships are enriched by all of the parts of a relationship: talking together, working together, facing trouble together, making love together. A strong relationship can survive having things put aside for a while but not for a long time. It is important that you find the time and energy to sustain a good relationship. Carefully review the discussion in Chapter 13. Make yourself find ways to create the romance and privacy you need at times when neither of you is exhausted.

## THE FUTURE

It is important that you plan for the future. The future will bring changes for the person with a dementing illness and many of these changes will be less painful if you are prepared for them.

Some husbands and wives discuss the future while both of

them are well. If you can do this, you will feel more comfortable going on by yourself, knowing what your partner wished for you. If she wishes to do so, the forgetful person may talk about the future when she is unable to care for herself or after her death. Planning how she will dispose of her possessions sometimes helps a person to feel that this is her life, and that she has some control over the end of her life. Other people will not want to think about these things and should not be pressured to do so.

Members of the family may also want to discuss what the future will bring, talking it over, perhaps a little at a time. Sometimes, thinking about the future is to painful for some members of the family. If this happens, you may have to plan alone.

Here are some of the things you will want to consider. (We have discussed each of these concerns elsewhere in this book.)

What will the ill person be like as his illness progresses and as he becomes increasingly physically disabled?

What kind of care will he need?

How much will you honestly be able to continue to give to this person?

At what point will your own emotional resources be exhausted?

What other responsibilities do you have that must be considered?

Do you have a spouse, children, or a job that also demands your times and energies?

What effect will this added burden have on your marriage, on growing children, or on your career?

Where can you turn for help?

How much help will the rest of the family give you?

What financial resources are available for this person's care?

What will be left for you to live on after you have met the expenses of care? It is important to make financial plans for the future even if you and the ill person have only a limited income. The care of a severely ill person can be expensive. (See Chapter 15.)

What legal provisions have been made for this person's care?

Will the physical environment make it difficult for you to care for an invalid?

Do you live in a house with stairs that the person will eventually be unable to manage? Do you live in a big house that may be difficult to maintain? Do you live a long way from stores? Do you live in an area where crime is a problem?

As time passes, you, the caretaker, may change. In some ways you may not be the same person you were before this illness. You may have given up friends and hobbies because of this illness, or you may have changed your philosophy or your ideas in the process of learning to accept this chronic illness. What will your future be like? What should you do to prepare for it?

## You as a Spouse Alone

This was a difficult section of this book for us to write. We know that husbands and wives think about their futures but we have no "right" answers to give you. Each person is unique. What is right for one person is not right for another, and only you can make those decisions. However, as you think through these things, there are several factors you will want to consider.

Your status changes. Sometimes a spouse feels that she is neither part of a couple (because they cannot still do things together, still talk together, and still rely on each other in the same ways) nor a widow.

Couples sometimes find that friends drift away from them. This is a particularly difficult problem for the well partner. "Couple" friends often drift away simply beause the friendship was based on the relationship among four people which has now changed. Establishing new friendships can be difficult when you can no longer include your spouse and yet you still have the responsibility for his care. You may not want to make new friends alone.

You may face a future without the ill person. Statistics indicate that dementing illnesses shorten the life of the victim. It is probable that she will die before you do or that she will become so ill that she needs nursing home care.

It is important that when the time comes that you are alone, you have friends and interests of your own.

*A husband told of trying to write an account of what it is like to live with a person suffering from a dementing illness. He said, "I realized that I was telling the story of my own deterioration. I gave up my job to take care of her, then I had no time for my hobbies, and gradually we stopped seeing our friends."*

As the illness progresses and the person needs more and more care, you may find yourself giving up more and more of your own life in order to care for her. Friends do drift away, there is no time for hobbies, and you can find youself alone with an invalid.

What then happens to you after she has become so ill that she must be placed in a nursing home or after she dies? Will you have "deteriorated"—become isolated, without other interests, lonely, used up? You need your friends and your hobbies through the long illness to give yourself support and a change of pace from the job of care giver. You are going to need them very much after you are left alone.

The marital relationship between husband and wife changes. The problems of being alone but not single are real. However, the relationship usually continues to have meaning. For some this means a continuing commitment to a changed relationship. For some it means establishing a new relationship with another person.

*One husband said, "I will always take care of her but I've started dating again. She is no longer the person I married."*

*A wife says, "It was a terribly difficult decision. For me, the guilt was the hardest part."*

*Another husband said, "For me, caring for her, keeping my promise, is most important. It is true that she is not the same, but this too is a part of our marriage. I try to see it as a challenge."*

Sometimes it happens that a person falls in love again while he is still caring for his ill spouse. If this happens to you, you face difficult decisions about your own beliefs and values. Perhaps you will want to talk this over with other people close to you. Perhaps the "right" decision is the decision that is "right" for you.

Not all marriages have been happy. When a marriage was so unhappy that a spouse was already considering divorce when the person became ill, the illness can make the decision more difficult. A good counselor can help you sort out your mixed feelings.

In any event, should you be faced with questions about new relationships, divorce, or remarriage, you are not alone. Many others have also faced—and resolved—these things.

# 13

## CARING FOR YOURSELF

THE SICK PERSON'S well-being depends directly on your well-being. *It is essential that you find ways to care for yourself so that you will not exhaust your own emotional and physical resources.*

When you care for a person who has a dementing illness, you may feel sad, discouraged, frustrated, or trapped. You may be tied or overburdened. While there are many reasons for feeling fatigued, the most common is not getting enough rest. You may put aside your own needs for rest, friends, and time alone in order to care for the sick person.

Throughout this book we have offered suggestions for ways to modify annoying behaviors. While modifying the person's behavior will help considerably, it is often not possible to eliminate some behaviors and they may continue to get on your nerves. In order to continue to cope, you will need to get enough rest and sometimes to get away from the ill person.

It is not unusual for family members to feel alone in their struggle with a chronic illness. Friends drift away and one doesn't know about other people with similar problems. It may seem impossible to get out of the house, and life narrows down to a tight circle of lonely misery. Feelings of sadness and grief seem more painful when you also feel alone with your problem.

For all of these reasons you need to take care of yourself. You need enough rest, time away from the sick person, and friends to enjoy, to share your problems with, and to laugh with. You may find that you need additional help to cope with your feelings of discouragement or to sort out the disagreements in the family. You may decide that it will help you to join other families to exchange concerns, to make new friends, and to advocate better resources for people with dementing illnesses.

## TAKE TIME OUT

*"If only I could get away from 'Alzheimer's disease,'"* Mrs. Murray said. *"If only I could go someplace where I didn't have to think about 'Alzheimer's disease' for a little while."*

It is absolutely essential—both for you and for the person with a dementing illness—that you have regular times to "get away" from twenty-four-hour care of the chronically ill person. You must have some time to rest and to be able to do some things *just for yourself*. This might be sitting down uninterrupted to watch TV or it might be sleeping through the night. It may mean going out once a week or taking a vacation. We cannot overemphasize the importance of this. The continued care of a person with a dementing illness can be an exhausting and emotionally draining job. It is quite possible to collapse under the load.

It is important that you have other people to help you, to

talk with, and to share your problems. We know that it can be difficult to find ways to care for yourself. You may not have understanding friends, your family may not be willing to help, and it may seem impossible to get time away from the sick person. The confused person may refuse to stay with anyone else, or you may not be able to afford help. Finding ways to meet your own needs often takes effort and ingenuity. However, it is so important that it must be done.

If resources to give you time out are difficult to find, perhaps you can piece together a respite plan. For example,

*Mr. Cooke persuaded the day care center to take his wife one day a week by agreeing to teach the staff how to manage her. His son, who lived out of state, agreed to pay for the day care. His neighbors agreed to come over and help get his wife dressed on those mornings.*

You may also have to compromise and accept a plan that is not as good as you would like. The care others give may not be the same as the care you try to give. The confused person may be upset by the changes. Family members may complain about being asked to help. Paying for care may mean financial sacrifices. But be persistent in your search for help, and be willing to piece things together and to make compromises.

Taking time out, away from the care of the confused person, is one of the single most important things that you can do to make it possible for you to continue to care for someone with a dementing illness.

*Mrs. Murray went on, "We had planned for a long time to go to France when he retired. When I knew he would never be able to go, I went alone. I left him with my son. I was scared to go alone, so I went with a tour group. He would have wanted me to, and when I came back I was rested— ready to face whatever came next."*

## Give Yourself a Present

Could you use a "lift" once in a while? An occasional self-indulgence is another way to help yourself cope. Some people may buy themselves "presents"—a magazine or a new dress. Listen to a symphony or the ballgame (use earphones), stand outside and watch the sunset, order your favorite restaurant as a carry out.

## Friends

Friends are often marvelously comforting, supportive, and helpful. The support of good friends will do much to keep you going through the hardest times. Remember that it is important for you to continue to have friends and social contacts. Try not to feel guilty about maintaining or establishing friendships on your own.

Sometimes friends and neighbors find it hard to accept that a person is ill when he *looks* fine. Sometimes, too, people shy away from "mental" illnesses. Many people do not know how to act around a person who is forgetful or whose behavior changes. You may want to explain that this is an organic disease that causes gradual deterioration of the mind. The person cannot help his behavior and he is not "crazy" or "psychotic." There is no evidence that the disease is contagious. It is a disease condition and not the inevitable result of old age.

Even if the person can talk quite reasonably, and a casual observer cannot see any sign of mental deterioration, he may still not be remembering names or really following conversations. It is important to explain to friends that forgetfulness is not bad manners but something the person cannot avoid.

It can be painful to tell old friends what is happening, especially those who do not live nearby and have not seen the gradual changes a dementing disease causes. Some families have solved this problem by composing a Christmas letter, lovingly and honestly sharing this illness with distant friends.

## Avoid Isolation

What can you do if you find yourself becoming isolated? It takes energy and effort to make new friends at a time when you may be feeling tired and discouraged. But this is so important that you must make the necessary effort. Start by finding one small resource for yourself. Little things will give you the guidance and energy to find others. Join a discussion group for families or get one going yourself. Renew ties with your church or synagogue. Your rabbi, priest, or minister can offer you comfort and support. Friendships within the church can develop, and many churches have some resources to provide practical help for you.

As you find time for yourself away from the person you are caring for, use that time to do things with other people: pursue a hobby or attend discussion groups. New friends are most easily made when you are involved in activities you have in common with other people.

We know that it is difficult to find the time or energy to do anything beyond the necessary care of the sick person. Some activities can be put on the "back burner" while you are burdened with care, but they must not be completely discontinued. This is important. When the time comes that you no longer have the care of this person, you will need friends and activities.

*"I like to go to the Masonic Lodge. I still go once a month. When Alice has to go to a nursing home, I'll probably get more involved—volunteer to run the Christmas drive or something. I still have my friends there."*

*"I play a violin. I can't play with the quartet anymore, but I keep in touch with them and I still practice a little.*

*When I have more time, there will be a place for me in the community symphony."*

You may also become involved in new activities, such as joining a local Alzheimer's organization. Some spouses have deliberately sought out new activities.

*"My wife got sick just about the same time I retired. All I was doing was taking care of her. I thought I should get some exercise, so I joined a senior citizens' exercise group. I take my wife to a day care center the day I go to that group."*

## FIND ADDITIONAL HELP IF YOU NEED IT

*Mrs. Scott says, "I worry that I am drinking too much. John and I used to have a cocktail when he got home in the evening. Now, of course, he doesn't drink, but I find I have to have that cocktail and another one at bedtime."*

Fatigue, discouragement, anger, grief, despair, guilt, and ambivalence are all normal feelings that may come with caring for a chronically ill person. Such feelings may seem overwhelming and almost constant. The burden you carry can be staggering. Sometimes one's coping skills are overwhelmed and things can drift out of control. You may want to seek professional help if this happens.

### Recognize the Warning Signs

Each individual is different and each person has his own ways of responding to problems. A healthy response for one person may be unhealthy for another. Ask yourself the following questions: Do I feel so sad or depressed that I am not functioning as I should? Am I often lying awake at night worrying? Am I losing weight? Do I feel overwhelmed most of the time? Do I feel terribly isolated and alone with my problem? While depression and discouragement are common feelings for families of people with chronic diseases, if you are often lying awake at night worrying, if you are losing weight, or if you usually feel isolated, alone with your problem, or overwhelmed, perhaps you need some help to keep your feelings manageable.

Am I drinking too much? Definitions of alcohol abuse vary widely. The amount of alcohol that is too much for one person may not be too much for another. Ask yourself: Is my drinking interfering with how I function with my family, or my job, or in other ways? If it is, you are drinking too much. Are you ever drinking too much to care properly for the sick person? Are others—your co-workers, for example—having to "cover" for you? Alcoholics Anonymous (listed in the telephone directory) is a good self-help organization. Often the group will help you solve the practical problems like transportation and finding a "sitter" so that you can get to the meetings. Call them, explain your special circumstances, and ask for their assistance.

Am I using pills to get me through each day? Tranquilizers and sleeping pills should be used only under the careful supervision of a physician and only for a short time. Pep pills (amphetamines) should never be used to give you an energy boost. If you are already using tranquilizers, sleeping pills, or pep pills on a regular basis, ask a doctor to help you give them up. Some of these drugs create a drug dependency. Abrupt withdrawal can be life-threatening and must be supervised by a doctor.

Suppose you are abusing alcohol or medications. You have joined the ranks of thousands of other ordinary people. There is no reason to be ashamed. There *is* a reason to get help *now*.

Am I drinking too much coffee each day? While nowhere near as serious as amphetamine abuse, excessive caffeine use can be hard on your body and can reduce your ability to manage stress. (Caffeine is also found in tea and most soft drinks.)

Am I screaming or crying too much? Am I often losing my temper with the impaired person? Am I hitting him? Do I find myself more angry and frustrated after I talk with my friends or family about these problems? Do I find that I am getting irritated with a lot of people—friends, my family, the doctors, my coworkers—more than just one or two people in my life?

How much screaming or crying is too much? One person may feel that any crying is too much, while another feels that crying is a good way to "get things out of my system." You probably know already if your moods are exceeding what is normal for you.

Anger and frustration are normal responses to caring for a person whose behavior is difficult. However, when your anger begins to spill over into many relationships or when yu take your anger out on the sick person, it may be helpful to find ways to manage your frustrations so that it does not drive people away from you or make the impaired person's behavior worse.

Am I thinking about suicide?

*Mr. Cameron said, "There was a time when I considered getting a gun, killing my wife, and then killing myself."*

The thought of suicide can come when a person is feeling overwhelmed, helpless, and alone. When someone feels that he cannot escape an impossible situation or when someone feels that he has irrevocably lost the things that make life worth living, he may consider suicide. Suicide may be considered when someone feels that the situation he faces is hopeless, when he feels that there is nothing either he or anyone else can do. The present can seem intolerable, and the future appears bleak, dark, empty, and meaningless.

*One family member who attempted suicide said, "Looking back, I don't know why I felt that way. Things have been hard, but I'm glad I didn't die. My perceptions must have been all mixed up."*

This consideration—that one's perception is that things are hopeless—is important. If you are feeling this way, it is important to find another person (a counselor, if possible) whose perception of the situation may be different and with whom you can talk.

Do I feel that I am out of control of my situation or at the end of my rope? Is my body telling me I am under too much stress? Do I often feel panicky, nervous, or frightened? Would it help just to talk the whole thing over with someone who understands? If the answer to some of these questions is yes, it may be that you are carrying too heavy a burden without enough help.

## Counseling

It may be that all you need is more time away from a seemingly demanding, difficult person or more help in caring for him. But perhaps you see no way to find more help or more time for yourself. Perhaps you see yourself trapped by your situation. We feel that talking these problems over with a trained person is one good way to help you feel less pressured. You and he can sort out the problems you face a bit at a time. Since he is not as caught up in the problem as you are, he may be able to see workable alternatives you had not thought of. At the same time you will know that you have a life line in this person that you can turn to when you begin to feel desperate. Family or friends can be of help as well, but if they are too close to the situation they may not be able to see things objectively.

Should you get counseling? Do you need "help"? Most people are not "sick," "crazy," or "neurotic." Most people are healthy individuals who sometimes have trouble coping with real problems. They may feel overwhelmed or discouraged, or find that they are thinking in circles. Such a person may find that talking over feelings and problems helps to clarify them.

We believe that most people most of the time do not need counseling. However, we know that counseling is sometimes a great help to families struggling with a dementing illness. Such help may come from discussion groups, clergy, an objective friend, or a social worker, nurse, psychologist, or physician.

The first step in seeking outside help is often the hardest. One's reasoning sometimes goes around and around in circles.

*"I can't get out of the house because I can't get a sitter. He's terrible to anyone in the house but me. I can't afford counseling because I can't get a job because I can't leave the house and a counselor couldn't help me with that anyway."*

This kind of circular thinking is partly the product of your situation and partly the way you, in your discouragement, see the problem. A good counselor can help you objectively separate the problem into more manageable parts, and together you can begin to make changes a little at a time.

Sometimes people feel that it is a sign of their own weakness or inadequacy to go to a counselor. With the burden you carry in coping with a dementing illness, you can use all the help you can get, and this is not a reflection on your strength.

People sometimes avoid counseling because they think that the therapist will delve into their childhood and "analyze" them. Many therapists begin directly by helping you in a matter-of-fact way to cope with "here and now" concerns. Find out in advance what approach the therapist you select prefers. If you decide to seek counseling, the kind of counselor you choose may be influenced by what you can afford, who is available, and who is knowledgeable about dementing illnesses.

Psychiatrists are physicians and they are able to prescribe drugs to treat mental illness. They have a good understanding of physical problems that accompany psychological problems. Psychologists, social workers, psychiatric nurses, clergy, and some other professionals can have excellent therapeutic or counseling skills. If they do, they may be an excellent choice for counseling. You will want to select a person whose services you can afford, who is knowledgeable about dementing illnesses, and with whom you feel comfortable.

You have a responsibility to discuss with the counselor your concerns about your relationship with him. If you are worried about your bill, if you don't like his approach, if you wonder if he is telling your family what you have said, *ask* him.

There are several ways to find a counselor. If you have an established relationship with a clergyman or a physician with whom you feel comfortable, ask if he can counsel you or can refer you to someone he feels is a good counselor. If you have friends who have had counseling, ask them if they liked the person they consulted. If there is an active family group in your area, ask if there is someone other members have consulted.

If you cannot find someone through such recommendations, counseling services or referral are available from the community mental health clinic or from religious-affiliated service agencies like Jewish Family and Children's Society, Associated Catholic Charities, or Pastoral Counseling Services (these agencies usually serve people of all religions). The county medical society can give you the names of local psychiatrists.

Not all counselors are equally good, nor are they all knowledgeable about dementia. Select a counselor as carefully as you would any other service you seek and know what

his credentials as a therapist are. If, after a period of time,
you do not think the counselor is helping you, discuss this
with him and then consider trying a different therapist.

## JOINING WITH OTHER FAMILIES:
## A STEP BEYOND

Many families feel alone with this illness, unable to find
doctors, other professionals, or friends who understand, and
unable to get information. To meet this need for communication,
families in many areas have established volunteer organizations.
These groups are involved in helping each other, sharing
solutions to management problems, exchanging information,
supporting needed legislation and research, and educating the
community. These organizations welcome members who are
concerned about all of the dementing illnesses, of which
Alzheimer's disease is the most common. Over and over, all
over the country, families tell us how important it is to know
other families who are faced with these problems. The number of family support groups is growing rapidly. These groups
offer friendship, information about the disease, and information about resources and doctors in your area, and they give
their members the opportunity to exchange ideas about how to
manage.

These volunteer organizations across the country have established a national organization, the Alzheimer's Disease and
Related Disorders Association (ADRDA), whose goals include family support, education, advocacy, and encouraging
research. (The address for the national association is listed in
Appendix 2.) The national organization will give you the
address of local groups near you. If there is no family group
near you, they will give you the names of other family
members you can talk to. Some other family members
generously offer friendship and support over the telephone.
Just talking to another person may help enormously.

Some organizations publish newsletters that may be helpful to you even if you live too far away to attend meetings. Newsletters give ideas on how to cope, notices of changes in legal policies and insurance coverage, and news about new research.

It is through organization that legislative attention will be focused on the needs of families and patients.

## SETTING UP AN ORGANIZATION OR SUPPORT GROUP

If no group exists near you, consider forming one yourself. Start out by finding three or four other families and perhaps a helpful professional (a minister, social worker, or nurse). It is not hard to find other families. Word of mouth will probably turn up three or four. Local ministers, nursing homes, visiting nurse associations, social workers, and the Office on Aging can put you in touch with others.

Your group can begin by writing for information from other groups and my informally exchanging ideas. Here are some suggestions for setting up a support group:

1. At the first meeting, establish specific time limits for meetings and stick to them. Meetings that run late may become a burden. For the same reason, if refreshments are served, agree to keep them simple.
2. Set simple, specific objectives for each meeting. These could be "informal discussion of problems" or "electing officers," but objectives will help keep the group on target.
3. Avoid tackling too much at a time. A few concrete, attainable goals are less likely to overwhelm people already under pressure in their private lives.
4. Be informed. Find out what other groups are going.
5. Discuss the members' responsibility to maintain confidentiality about personal information shared in the group.

6. Different people have different ways of reacting to crisis. Make it clear from the start that members will not be judgmental.
7. Agree to let each person have time to talk, so that no one person dominates the conversation.

Family members who are caring for a sick person at home may have little energy left over for the work of organizing a group. Some families whose loved one has entered a nursing home or has died are happy to participate and will be a resource to the group. Also, professionals who work with the elderly may wish to join the group and can lend their skills to help keep the group going. Local community colleges, service organizations, county extension offices, and churches may be willing to sponsor a group. They may also have staff with expertise in setting up volunteer organizations.

The Alzheimer's Disease and Related Disorders Association has a kit for new groups. You can obtain it from them.

## Sharing Groups

Many organizations and hospitals have established discussion groups for family members. These are small sharing groups led by a trained therapist. Families find these groups helpful. Such groups can be set up by anyone with skills in group therapy. Guidelines for professionals establishing groups are available in the gerontology literature (see Appendix 1).

## Peer Support Groups

Lay support groups sometimes operate without professional guidance. Such groups should have goals of mutual encouragement and not be used as therapy groups. They should consist of four to ten people. One way to handle leadership is to met each time at a different home. The discussion leader for that meeting is the host, thus rotating leadership through the group. It is often helpful for members to make a commitment to regular participation for a certain set number of meetings. At the first meeting, discuss items 1, 5, 6, and 7 listed previously under "Setting Up a Group." In addition, remember that this is not a therapy group; it is a group for mutual exchange and support. Give each person present an opportunity to talk. One or two people should not monopolize the discussion. Good group members avoid giving each other advice. Instead, they listen with interest and concern and give information.

## ADVOCACY AND ACTIVISM

Throughout this book we have emphasized the need for resources to help you. However, the unfortunate fact is that resources you need may not be available, physicians and other professionals are often not informed about dementing illnesses, state and federal governments and insurance companies often have regulations that discriminate against people with dementia, and funding for patient care and research may not be available. It has been estimated that 2 million Americans are impaired with a dementing illness and an additional 2 million may suffer from mild cognitive impairment. Clearly, the prevailing lack of interest in these diseases and the assumption that "senility" is not even a disease is unfounded and unjust and leads to discriminatory regulations.

Only when the public and the policy makers recognize that dementias are diseases and become aware of the needs of the patients and families will new resources and adequate funding be made available. You may want to do what you can to urge that new or better resources be developed, or that unjust policies be changed. You may want to help to educate those who are not informed about dementia. Here are some ways in which to make your efforts most effective:

1. Discuss your opinion with your state and federal legislators and ask what you can do to support change. Give

them your specific concerns in writing. Write to legislators, the state Office on Aging, the National Council on Aging, and national senior citizen organizations and express your concerns.

2. Act as a group with other families of people with dementing illnesses. Contact the Alzheimer's Disease and Related Disorders Association. Contact and work with an advocacy group such as the Gray Panthers (address in Appendix 2).

3. Give written information and bibliographies about these problems to the people, including physicians, with whom you have contact. Libraries have materials with specific guidelines for effective activism that you can use to make your voice most effective.

# 14

## For Children And Teenagers

This chapter is written especially for the young people who live with or know a person with a dementing illness. Most young people will be able to read and understand the rest of the book as well.

It is important that you understand what is wrong with the person and why he acts as he does. When you understand why the person does certain things, it is easier not to get mad at him. Also, it is important that you understand that he acts as he does because he is sick, not because he wants to or because of you. The person has a disease that destroys part of the brain. With a larger number of brain cells lost, the brain cannot work as it should. That is why the person forgets names, is clumsy, or can't talk properly. Parts of the brain that knew how to do these things have been damaged.

Sometimes these people get upset over little things. That is because the brain can no longer understand what is going on (even when you explain to the person). The parts of the brain that make us behave as we should are also damaged, so the person cannot control his actions. He cannot help himself. Sometimes people with dementing illnesses don't look sick or act strange, but they may criticize you or correct you too much. The person may not be able to help this because his illness makes him forget things.

You may worry about what will happen to the person or about whether something you do might make him worse, especially when you are not sure what is happening. Most likely nothing you can do will make the person worse. You can make him temporarily more upset, but this does not make his condition worse.

If you worry about things, ask questions. Read other parts of the book. You may want to go back to it from time to time. Read any other material you can find on these diseases also. Ask your parents or the doctor treating the person what you want to know. You will get the best results if you bring the subject up when there are not a lot of other things going on and when the adults are not too tired. However, sometimes adults try to keep bad news from young people.

When you read or talk about these diseases, what you find out may be bad news. The person may not be going to get well. You may react by feeling bad about the whole thing. If there are things you really don't want to know, don't feel that you are expected to ask about them. Many people have mixed feelings—you may feel sorry for the sick person but also angry that he has to live at your house. Your moods may change a lot too. Sometimes you may put the whole thing out of your mind and not even be able to think about it. Most of these reactions are the normal result of facing problems.

Even under the best circumstances, living with an illness like this is hard. Here are some of the things that young people have told us are problems.

*"No privacy: Granddad walks into my room whenever he wants."*

*"Having to be quiet. Not being able to play the stereo. As soon as I come in the door I have to get quiet or Granddad gets excited."*

*"The way he eats makes me sick."*

*"I can't bring my friends over because they upset Granddad. Also, I don't want to bring them over because he acts so crazy."*

*"Having to give up my room."*

*"Everybody depends on me more. I have to take a lot of responsibility."*

*"Everybody is so busy with Granddad and so tired, we never do anything fun as a family anymore."*

*"I'm afraid of what he will do."*

*"I'm afraid he will die."*

*"I just feel discouraged all the time."*

*"My parents get mad at me more than they used to."*

You may have some of the same concerns as these. You may be stuck with some problems, like having to be quiet or having to give up your room. Some things are easier when you understand what is wrong with the person. You can't cope with some things alone and you may need to get an adult to help you. Sometimes it is helpful to pick out the one thing that bothers you the most and ask your family to help you change that. Often, together you can come up with compromises that will help. For example, you might be able to put a lock on your door or get earphones for your stereo. If you have given up your room, perhaps you and your friends can fix up a place in the basement where you can get away from the sick person.

Some young people tell us that it is not the sick person's behavior that is the worst problem, but it is how their parents or the sick person's husband or wife acts that is the worst problem.

*"I don't mind Granddad, but Grandmother moved in too, and she wants me to do everything like she did when she was young."*

*"It isn't Granddad, it's my mother always fighting with my grandmother."*

These may be real problems for you. The person who is your grandparent is also a wife or husband of a sick person and is probably upset. Even when a person doesn't get upset he may be feeling sad or unhappy, and this may make that person cross or impatient or hard to live with. Probably the best you can do is to be understanding, since you know that grief and worry are the causes of the trouble. When a grandparent is setting strict standards for you or nagging you, ask your parents to tell you how they want you to handle this. If things get too difficult, find an adult who is not tired and upset—perhaps somebody outside your family—whom you can talk it over with.

Most of what we have written has been for people whose grandparent is sick, because usually people's children are grown before they develop a dementing illness. However, sometimes this illness strikes one's own parents. If it is your father or mother who is sick, things are probably really hard. We hope this book will help you. However, no book can solve problems that are happening in *your* house with *your* family.

It is important for you and your well parent to talk about what is happening and the problems you are having. In addition, it may be helpful for you, your well parent, and any other children in the family to find someone with whom you can all talk from time to time. If your well parent is unable to seek help, you may have to ask the doctor or your teachers to help you. No one with a parent who has a dementing illness should have to cope by himself.

Belonging to a scout troop or a church youth club or an athletic team or some other group will give you a chance to get away from the troubles at home and to get your mind on having fun with other young people.

Things are not all bad when a person has a dementing illness. Young people often have clever ideas about how to solve problems that the rest of the family may not have thought of. Also, perhaps because not too long ago you were little, you probably have a lot of understanding for the person who is confused. You will probably do a lot of growing up during this time and you may look back on it with pride.

It is important to remember, when you are caught in a situation you cannot control, that you *do* have control over how you react to it. You decide how a bad situation affects your life.

If your grades at school drop, or if you are fighting with your parents a lot or "tuning out" most of the time, you need to talk the problem over with someone. Often you can talk things over with your parents, other adult friends, or teachers. Some people are easy to talk to and some are not. Sometimes a counselor is a good person to talk with. If you cannot talk to your parents, your teachers can usually help you find a counselor. Some people feel funny about talking to a counselor. It isn't because there is something "wrong" with you that you get counseling. Here are some of the things that happen with a good counselor or someone else who is a good listener.

You can find out what's going on.

You can let off steam.

You can talk with your parents with the counselor helping so that you don't fight with them.

You can find out what your parents are thinking.

You can say all you want about your side.

You can ask about things that worry you—like whether the sick person will die—in private.

None of these things may solve the problem, but they will make living with the problem easier.

# 15

## FINANCIAL AND LEGAL ISSUES

To DISCUSS IN DETAIL the financial and legal issues that may arise around the care of a person with a dementing illness is beyond the purpose and scope of this book. However, we have outlined some of the key factors for you to consider. You may need to seek professional financial and legal advice.

### YOUR FINANCIAL ASSESSMENT

Providing care for the person with a chronic illness can be costly. In addition, the older person may be living on a fixed income and inflation can be expected to continue to eat into that income. It is important that you assess both financial resources and potentially increasing costs of care, and make plans for the impaired person's financial future. If you are a spouse, your own financial future may well be affected by decisions and plans you make now. Many factors must be considered in assessing your financial future, including the nature of the illness and your individual expectations.

Begin by assessing the potential costs of care both now and as the person becomes more severely impaired and by assessing her available resources. Whether the ill person has little income or is affluent, it is most important that you plan ahead for her financial future.

## Potential Expenses

*Potential lost income:*
Will the impaired person have to give up her job?

Will someone who would otherwise be employed have to stay at home to care for the person?

Will the impaired person lose retirement or disability benefits?

Will the real purchasing power of a fixed income decline as inflation rises?

*Potential housing costs:*
Will you or the impaired person have to move to a home that is without stairs, closer to services, or easier to maintain?

Will you move a parent into your home? This may mean expenses of renovating a room for her.

Will the person enter a life care facility, foster care, or sheltered housing?

Will you have to make modifications to your home (new locks, grab rails, safety devices, wheel chair ramps)?

*Potential medical costs:*
Will you need
   visiting nurses?
   doctors?
   medical insurance?
   evaluations?
   occupational therapists? physical therapists?
   medications?
   appliances (hospital bed, special chair, wheelchair)?

*Potential cost of help or respite care:*
Will you need
   someone to clean?

276

someone to stay with the person?
someone to help with care?
day care?
*Potential food costs:*
Will there be costs of having meals prepared or of eating out?
*Transportation costs:* (someone to drive if you cannot; taxis)
*Taxes:*
*Legal fees:*
*Miscellaneous costs:*
(Easy-to-use clothing, ID bracelets, incontinence supplies, diaper service, various devices for safety or convenience may be listed here.)
*Nursing home costs:*

## Potential Resources

### *The Impaired Person's Resources*

You will want to look first at the sick person's own assets and financial resources. Consider pensions, Social Security, savings accounts, real estate, automobiles, and any other potential sources of income or capital.

Occasionally, an impaired person becomes secretive about her finances. At the end of this chapter we list some of the possible available resources and where to look for them.

### *Resources of the Impaired Person's Spouse, Children, and Other Relatives*

(Also see Chapter 11.)

Laws regarding the financial rights and responsibilities of family members are complex and not all social workers or lawyers are completely familiar with them. (Also read pages 294–300 on financing nursing home care.)

In some cases (such as with Social Security), a divorced spouse may be entitled to benefits from a former husband or wife.

In some cases, the law differentiates between the rights of husbands and the rights of wives. Such laws are being rewritten in some states and may be declared invalid if tested in court.

It is important to know about laws that may affect a well spouse if the ill spouse may eventually need expensive care. Advance estate planning may protect the spouse financially. This is important for families of modest means as well as for more affluent families.

## Resources from Insurance

Health insurance and major medical insurance may help to pay for home care or needed appliances as well as for hospitalization, physicians' services, and medications. Health insurance policies often contain exclusions that affect payment for dementing or chronic illnesses. You need to know exactly what your insurance covers.

Find out what life insurance policies the person has and whether these can be a resource. Some insurance policies waive the premiums if the insured becomes disabled. This is a savings for her.

If you are eligible for Medicare (see p. 294), find out what it will pay for. Medicare will pay for some things that you may not have thought of and does not pay for other things that many families assume are covered. The laws and regulations governing what Medicare will cover occasionally change. If you were denied payment for something in the past, it may be worth your while to inquire again a year later if you still need the same thing.

Medicaid (see p. 296) is a federal program administered by the individual states. It provides for medical care for people who receive income from programs such as Supplemental Security Income or financial assistance programs. Other families who have high medical expenses may qualify for Medicaid. It pays for hospitalizations, physician visits, medications, and some kinds of health care. In some states, other services are also paid for. Families who have large medical bills should inquire about this resource from a social worker or the Department of Social Services.

## *Tax Breaks for the Elderly or for the Care of a Person with a Dementing Illness*

The elderly are eligible for various tax breaks. General information about this is in the Internal Revenue Service publication "Tax Benefits for Older Americans."

Tax deductions for the care of a person with a dementing illness can make a significant difference to families. You are entitled to medical deductions for someone who is your dependent. The definition of whom you may claim as your dependent for medical deductions and the tax credit for disabled dependents allow you to claim some people who might not otherwise qualify as your dependents.

If you work and must hire someone to care for your disabled dependent, you may be entitled to a tax credit for part of the cost of the care.

Some nursing home costs that are not covered by Medicare or Medicaid may be deductible. The definitions of what part of nursing home care can be deducted and when it can be deducted are complex, and you may want to review carefully the IRS and tax court definitions of whom you can claim as your dependent and what deductions you can take.

At the time of this writing, the tax laws are being examined by family organizations and some legislators who are urging tax relief for families who care for a disabled elderly person. You may want to look into the most recent legislation concerning your individual situation.

If you are uncertain about your rights, a tax consultant may be helpful to you. You do not have to accept as final the information given to you by the IRS staff.

## State, Federal, and Privately Supported Resources

State, federal, and private funds support a range of resources, such as day care centers, Meals-on-Wheels, food stamps, sheltered housing, mental health clinics, social work services, and recreation centers. The funding source usually defines the population to be served in specific terms (such as only people over sixty-five or people with income under a certain amount).

"Pilot" programs are programs funded for a brief period to determine their effectiveness.

"Research" programs are programs in which participants are studied in specific ways. Such programs sometimes offer excellent free or low-cost services. They usually have specific criteria for eligibility. Most research programs must meet exacting standards to assure that research does not harm the subjects. You will be asked to sign a consent form that explains exactly what research is being done, what risks, if any, are involved, and what benefits are to be expected. You also will be given the option of withdrawing from the study at any time.

## LEGAL MATTERS

(Also see Chapter 9.)

The time may come when a person with a dementing illness cannot continue to take legal or financial responsibility for herself. This may mean that she can no longer balance a checkbook or that she has forgotten what financial assets or debts she has. It may mean that she is unable to decide responsibly what to do with property or to give permission for needed medical care.

Often these abilities are not all lost at once. A person who is unable to manage her checkbook may still be able to make a will or accept medical care. However, as her impairment increases, she may gradually reach the point where she cannot make any decisions for herself, and someone else will have to assume legal responsibility for her.

The most efficient way to prepare for this eventual disability (which could happen to any of us) is for the person to make plans for herself *before* she reaches the time when she cannot do so. A person should make a will while she is still considered legally competent to do so. This is called *testamentary capacity.* It means that the person knows, without prompting, that she is making a will, the names of and her relationship to the people who will receive her property, and the nature and extent of the property.

A person who is still able to manage her own affairs (by the above definition) may sign a *power of attorney,* which gives a spouse, child, or any other person who has reached legal age authority to manage her property. A power of attorney can give broad authority to the specified person or it can be limited. A limited power of attorney only gives the person authority to do specific things (sell a house or review income tax records, for example). When a power of attorney is intended to authorize someone to act in behalf of a person who may become increasingly disabled, it must state that it can be exercised even if the person becomes disabled.

Since a power of attorney authorizes someone to act in another person's behalf, the person giving such power must be sure that the one selected will, in fact, act in her best interests. Someone who holds a power of attorney is legally responsible to act in the other person's best interests, but once in a while someone abuses this responsibility.

We believe that it is important to discuss with a lawyer what plans you should make, so that he can advise you on how best to protect the confused person and what type of powers should be transferred, and so that you can be sure that whatever papers are drawn up are legally valid.

By making a will and granting a power of attorney while she is still able to do so, the person who feels her memory may be beginning to fail can be sure that if she gets worse her life will continue the way she intended and her property be distributed as she wished, rather than in a way imposed by a court or by state law. The person may continue to manage her own affairs or part of them until such time as a designated person must take over. Then the appointed person will usually not need to take further steps before she is legally able to take over the management of the sick person's affairs.

Some people are unwilling to sign a power of attorney, have no one that they trust to do this, or may already be too impaired to do so. If this is so, you will need the help of an attorney. Ask a friend or family member to recommend one. If you do not know an attorney, you can call the state bar association (listed in the phone directory as Maryland Bar Association, California Bar Association, etc.). They can give you the names of lawyers near you. Lawyers specialize in different areas of law (criminal law, corporate law, divorce law, civil law), just as doctors specialize in different areas of medicine. You have a right to know what you can expect from the lawyer and what his fees are. Misunderstandings can be avoided by discussing with him what he charges and what services you will get for that fee. Find out if he practices this sort of law and is knowledgeable about it.

If the person is currently unable to manage her property and affairs effectively because of her disability, a *guardianship of property* procedure (also called a conservatorship) may be necessary. In this procedure, the lawyer must file a petition in court. After a hearing, a judge decides whether the person is legally competent to manage her property or financial affairs. The judge may appoint a legal guardian to act for the person in financial matters only. This guardian must file financial reports periodically with the court.

If a home is owned jointly by a husband and wife, and one of them becomes impaired, the well spouse will need a power of attorney or guardianship of the property in order to sell the home.

Sometimes a disabled person is unable to care for her daily needs and must have medical care or nursing hom care. She may refuse to consent to this or may be unable to make such decisions. Often a hospital or nursing home will accept the consent of the next of kin: a husband or wife, or a son or daughter. Sometimes, however, a petition must be filed in court to request a *guardianship of the person*. The judge may then appoint a guardian of the person, order the needed care, or send the person to a hospital. This procedure is more complex than filing for guardianship of the property. Often a guardianship of the person is not obtained when a spouse or other family member is caring for her.

## WHERE TO LOOK FOR THE FORGETFUL PERSON'S RESOURCES

Sometimes an impaired person forgets what financial resources she has or what debts she owes. People may be private about their resources or disorganized in recording them. Sometimes suspiciousness is a part of the illness and the individual hides what she has. Families may not know what resources a person has that could be used to provide for her care.

*A wife said, "I did not know the V.A. hospital would care for him. I was spending $1,500 a month for a nursing home I didn't like and I never even asked about V.A."*

Finding out what resources a person has can be difficult, especially when things are in disarray or are hidden.

Debts usually turn up on their own, often in the mail. Most businesses will be understanding if a debt or bill is not paid on time. When you do find a bill, call the company, explain the circumstances, and arrange with them how and when the bill will be paid. If the confused person is losing the mail, you may be able to have it held for you at the post office.

Assets may be harder to find. Review recent mail. Look in the obvious places such as a desk, an office, clothing, and other places where papers are kept. Look under the bed, in shoe boxes, in pockets of clothes, in old purses, in teakettles or other kitchen items, under rugs, and in jewelry boxes. One wife asked the grandchildren to join her in a "treasure hunt." The children thought of obscure places to look. Look for: bank statements, canceled checks, bank books, savings books, passbooks, or checkbooks; keys; address books; insurance policies; receipts; business or legal correspondence; or income tax records for the past four or five years (a spouse filing a joint return or a person possessing a power of attorney or guardianship of property can obtain copies from the Internal Revenue Service. The power of attorney must meet IRS standards or be on their form). These items can be used to piece together a person's resources.

There are many kinds of assets.

*Bank accounts.* Look for bank books, bank statements, checkbooks, savings books, passbooks, statements of interest paid, joint accounts held with others. Most banks will not release information about accounts, loans, or investments to anyone whose name is not on the account. However, they may give limited information (such as whether there is an account in an individual's name) if you send a letter to the bank from your doctor or lawyer explaining the nature of the person's disability and the reason you need the information. Banks will release information about the amount in an account or about current transactions only to a court-appointed guardian or other properly authorized person. However, often you can piece together what you need to know from papers you can find.

*Stock certificats, bonds, certificates of deposit, savings bonds, mutual funds.* Look for the actual bonds, notices of payments due, notices of dividends paid, earnings claimed on income tax, regular amounts paid out from a bank account, receipts. Mutual funds are accounts held in the name of the broker; look for canceled checks, correspondence, or receipts from a broker. Look for record of purchases or sale.

*Insurance policies* (life insurance, disability insurance, health insurance). These are among the most frequently overlooked assets. Life insurance policies and health insurance policies may pay lump sum or other benefits. Look for premium notices, policies, or canceled checks that give you the name of the insurer. Contact him for full information about the policy. Some insurers will release this information upon receipt of a letter from a physician or attorney; others will need proof of your legal right to information.

*Safe deposit boxes.* Look for a key, bill, or receipt. You will need a court order to be permitted to open the box.

*Military benefits.* Look for discharge papers, dog tags, old uniforms. Contact the military to determine what benefits are available to the person. Dependents of veterans may be eligible for benefits.

*Real estate property* (houses, land, businesses, rental property, joint ownership or partial ownership of the above). Look for regular payments into or from a checking account, gains or losses declared on income tax, keys, fire insurance premiums (on houses, barns, businesses, or trailers). The insurance agent may be able to help you. Look for property tax assessments. Ownership of real estate property is a matter of public record. The tax assessor's office may be able to help you locate properties if you have some clues.

*Retirement or disability benefits.* These are also often overlooked. You must apply for Social Security, SSI (Supplemental Security Income), veterans benefits, or railroad retirement if you are eligible. Spouses and divorced spouses may also be eligible for benefits. Federal and state government employees, union members, clergy, and military personnel may have special benefits. Check into retirement or disability benefits from *all* past employers. Look for an old job résumé, which will list previous jobs. Look for benefit letters.

*Collections, gold, jewelry, cash, loose gems, autos, antiques, art, boats, camera equipment, furniture, other negotiable property.* In addition to looking for such items, look for valuable items listed on property insurance policies. Some of these items are small enough to be easily hidden. Others may be in plain sight and so familiar as to be overlooked.

*Wills.* If the individual has made a will, it should list her assets. Wills, if not hidden, are often kept in a safe deposit box, recorded by the court, or kept by one's attorney.

*Trust accounts.* Look for statements of interest paid.

*Personal loans.* Look for withdrawals, payments, correspondence, alimony payments (occasionally divorce settlements provide for payment of alimony should the wife become disabled).

*Foreign bank accounts.* Look for statements of interest paid, bank statements.

*Inheritance.* Find out whether the impaired person is someone else's heir.

*Cemetery plot.* Look for evidence of purchase.

# 16

## NURSING HOMES AND OTHER LIVING ARRANGEMENTS

SOMETIMES A FAMILY IS to care for a person with a dementing illness at home, even if relief services are available. A number of other living arrangements may be considered. Sometimes a mildly impaired person can continue to live independently if he has some help. He may prefer this to moving in with your family. There are a variety of residential care facilities in which an elderly couple or individual can live and receive different degrees of help or services.

### SHOULD YOU MOVE?

We have discussed ways to help a confused person accept a move on p. 66.

Sometimes a care giver moves to a residence where he can manage the confused person more easily: an apartment or a retirement home, for example. If you are contemplating moving, there are several things you will want to consider:

1. The financial costs of moving, such as the cost of a new residence, moving costs, closing costs, and capital gains tax on property you sell.
2. Will moving mean less property for you to clean or maintain? Will help for you, such as meal preparation or house cleaning, be provided?
3. Will moving bring you closer to doctors, hospitals, shopping centrs, recreation areas?
4. What kind of transportation will you need?
5. Will moving make you closer to or further from friends and family who can help you?
6. Will moving affect your eligibility for special programs or financial assistance? If you have sold your house, you may be required to spend your capital on nursing home care before you are eligible for Medicaid. You are not usually required to sell a house in which you are living to pay for care (see p. 299). You may not be eligible for some programs until you have lived in the state for a given period of time.
7. Will moving provide a safe environment for the person (no stairs, call bells, a ground floor bathroom, supervision, lower crime rate)?

*Retirement villages* and *senior citizens' apartments or condominiums* are planned for retired people who can live independently. In a condominium, the resident pays for a mortgage plus a monthly condominium fee for services such as maintenance of buildings and grounds, recreation facilities, security systems, and transportation to shopping areas. In senior citizens' apartments, the resident pays rent. Retirement villages may be set up as rental units or as condominiums. These forms of housing may provide emergency call services and easy access to medical facilities, but they generally do not offer special help for confused or ill people.

Section 8 of the Housing and Urban Development Act

provides for *federal rent subsidies* to the low-income elderly and handicapped. Public housing with low rentals for people with low incomes may also be available. Transportation or recreation facilities may be nearby, but usually no facilities are provided for those who cannot function independently. There are usually waiting lists for this type of housing.

*Sheltered housing* provides apartments or rooms for people who cannot live independently but who do not need constant supervision. Many sheltered housing units have safety features such as grab bars, wheelchair ramps, and call bells. In addition to security systems and transportation, these programs often offer meals, social work assistance, and someone to check on residents regularly. Some have a nurse on the staff or a medical clinic in the building. People with dementing illnesses usually must be able to provide their own personal care and not be disruptive or wander. Sheltered housing is funded under several different programs, including Section 8 (HUD), and costs vary.

*Boarding or domiciliary homes* provide a room, some housekeeping, and meals for several elderly people. Fees range widely. Depending on the state, licensure and inspection of these homes can be strict, lax, or nonexistent. As state mental hospitals have moved to discharge elderly patients, these homes have proliferated as the only place these displaced people can go to live. Although some such homes are excellent and are run by caring people, you will want to scrutinize the quality of care a person in such a home actually receives.

*Church-run homes for the elderly* may be life care communities, they may provide residential or domiciliary care (that is, housekeeping, meals, and some personal care, but no medical or nursing care), or they may be nursing homes. Some are excellent. Most are nonprofit or charitable institutions.

*Life care facilities* provide, for an initial down payment or entrance fee plus a monthly fee, a living setting similar to that of a retirement village. As a person declines he will be moved within the facility to a sheltered or skilled nursing setting. Once the individual or couple are accepted, the facility may provide care for the rest of their life, even if the client runs out of money. These are often profit-making corporations. They invest your initial payment and, based upon actuarial data, can expect to make a profit before you die. The entrance fee for life care may be a fee for service and will not be returned to the client's estate. In other life care facilities the initial fee is a down payment for property which builds equity for the client's estate. Your state may have regulations governing these fees. These facilities may provide excellent care and this may be a wise investment.

In some states, *adult foster home programs* arrange for impaired people to live, for a fee, with a foster family. Such people are cared for as members of the family, and receive meals, a room, transportation to the doctor, social work assistance, and supervision. Depending on the program, these can be excellent or inadequate.

## EVALUATING A LIVING ARRANGEMENT

1. Be sure the physical plant is clean and safe (check the kitchen and bathroom).
2. Know what the costs are and what they cover. Ask about extra charges.
3. Know whether the staff understands dementing illnesses and how they care for people like the potential resident.
4. Determine how much and what kind of supervision, recreation, meals, transportation, social support, and medical support is available and whether this meets the confused person's needs.
5. Find out who will be responsible for the person's medications.
6. Review the requirements of licensure and find out how often inspections are carried out and by whom.

7. Find out what is done in case of a medical emergency.
8. Find out what fire alarms and evacuation plans exist.
9. Know under what conditions the resident would be asked to leave.
10. Carefully review the fine print of the contract. Ask a lawyer to help if you don't understand it.

Good care facilities of all kinds often have waiting lists. It is wise to look into possible alternatives well in advance of the time you may need them. This will enable you to get on a list and to assess how good a program really is. You can always stop the application process if you wish.

Good care costs money. Costs may be borne by the individual, charitable gifts, or tax funds. There is rarely enough money from any of these sources to provide quality care for all who need it.

Other people, whether they are foster care givers or life care staff, may do things differently from the way in which you would do them. You may need to accept the differences if you want the help. Also, remember that the forgetful confused person may give you an inaccurate report of what is happening.

## NURSING HOMES AND LONG-TERM CARE FACILITIES

As the disease progresses, it may become more difficult to care for a person at home. Taking care of a person with a dementing illness can be a twenty-four-hour-a-day job and may require the skills of a professionally trained individual. At some point the family may be unable to continue providing all the care that is needed.

Placing your family member in a nursing home can be a difficult decisions to make and it often takes time. Often families have tried everything else first. However, a time may come in the process of caring for a demented person when nursing home placement becomes the most responsible decision the family can make.

Family members may feel great sadness and grief at having to accept the inevitable decline of their spouse, parent, or sibling. Family members frequently have mixed feelings about nursing home placement. They may experience a sense of relief that a decision has finally been made and that part of the care will be assumed by others, and at the same time feel guilty for wanting someone else to take over these real burdens. Family members may feel angry that there are no other choices available to them.

Many people don't want to place a family member in a nursing home. They feel that they should care for their loved ones at home and they may have heard that American families "dump" unwanted old people in institutions. Not all families do care lovingly for their elderly members, but statistics clearly show that families are *not* dumping their elderly in nursing homes, that most families do all they can to postpone or prevent nursing home admissions, and that they *do not* abandon their elderly after placement. Instead, most families visit in the nursing home regularly.

We tend to think of the "good old days" as a time when families took care of their elderly at home. In fact, in the past not many people lived long enough for their families to be faced with the burden of caring for a person with a dementing illness. The people who did become old and sick were in their fifties and sixties and the sons and daughters who cared for them were considerably younger than you may be when your parent needs care in his seventies and eighties. Today many "children" of an ailing parent are themselves in their sixties or seventies.

The term *nursing home* brings negative images to many people's minds, but often nursing homes give good care and are the best alternative for an ill person. Some nursing homes do not give adequate care, and there has been much publicity about them. Not all homes, however, deserve a bad reputation, and this publicity has brought about needed changes that have mproved the quality of nursing home care.

It is not unusual for family members to disagree about nursing home plans. Some members of the family may want the impaired person to remain at home while others feel the time has come for him to enter a nursing home. It is helpful if all involved family members discuss the problem together. Misunderstandings and disagreements are often worse when everyone does not have all the facts. Everyone in the family should discuss at least these three topics: the cost of nursing home care and where that money is to come from (see p. 294), the characteristics of the home you select (see p. 302), and the changes that placement will make in each person's life.

Going to live in a nursing home is a major change for the afflicted person. His ability to respond to this change will be influenced by how ill he is. You will want to help him participate in this move and adjust to this change as much as he is able.

Once you have decided to look for nursing home care for someone, you will need to begin a four-step process:

1. Investigate all funding resources.
2. Have the ill person see a physician if he has not seen one recently. (Most homes require a recent medical exam.) It may also be necessary to obtain a ''level-of-care rating'' for the person.
3. Locate a suitable home.
4. Make the placement and adjust to the changes that the placement brings about for both you and the person who has moved to the nursing home.

## Paying for Care

Nursing home care is expensive. Before you can make a final decision, you need to know how much the care is going to cost, how this cost will be met, and whether meeting the cost will create a financial burden for members of the family.

There are several ways in which families can play for nursing home care. Some families or the sick person himself will be able to pay for the full cost of care. The patient may have private insurance that will pay part or all of the nursing home costs. Many insurance policies, however, contain exclusion clauses so that people with dementing illnesses are not covered.

If the person is a veteran, find out from the Veterans Administration to what extent they will be a resource for you. (Some families have had patients discharged from V.A. hospitals.)

In some cases, Medicare pays for part of nursing home care for a limited time period. However, in planning for nursing home placement, it is important not to overestimate Medicaid benefits. Medicare may pay for patients who do not have other resources.

### Medicare

Medicare is a federal program administered by the Health Care Financing Administration. Applications can be made through your local Social Security Office. Medicare is divided into parts A and B. The regulations are complex. It is important that you thoroughly explore what is available in your specific situation. What follows is general information, which may change.

People are eligible for Medicare part A if they are eligible for Social Security or Railroad Retirement and are sixty-five or over, or if they have received Social Security Disability for twenty-four months (people on disability need not be sixty-five). People who turned sixty-five before 1974 and are not eligible for Social Security may be eligible for Medicare part A and should inquire. People may purchase Medicare part A by paying a premium if they are sixty-five or older and are not eligible for Social Security.

People are eligible for Medicare part B if they are eligible for part A and if they pay the added premium.

Medicare covers a limited number of nursing home costs. It only pays for services in nursing homes certified as "skilled" facilities, meaning those that provide a relatively high level of nursing or rehabilitation care. To qualify for Medicare, the person must enter a nursing home following a hospital stay. Medicare recipients must need skilled nursing care or rehabilitation for the same condition for which they were treated in the hospital. "Skilled care" is defined by law and means that the patient needs the direct services or supervision of a registered nurse or licensed practical nurse or must qualify for rehabilitation services. If he needs skilled care, a person is entitled to twenty days of full coverage and eighty days of partial coverage. After that, other sources of funding must be found.

Sometimes people with dementing illnesses are denied Medicare for nursing home care because they are found to need "custodial" rather than skilled care. When a person does not need the care of a registered nurse or practical nurse (to review his medical status or to give injections, insert a catheter, etc.), but instead needs supervision (help with meals, help finding the bathroom, etc.), Medicare will not cover the cost. This clearly is unjust discrimination against people with dementing illnesses who need professional supervision to protect them from illness or injury. When a person needs only supervision, he may qualify if he needs a nurse to review his medical status daily. This is an important part of Medicare policy for people with dementing illnesses. (Also see page 198, which discusses Medicare coverage of home care.)

## Medicaid (Medical Assistance)

Medicaid is a program for which the patient or family must meet certain criteria. In general, one qualifies on the basis of the amount of income and assets (savings, property, etc.) that he has and on the basis of need. This is a federal program that is administered on the state level. Applications and information can be obtained through the local department of the agency that administers the program. This may be the Department of Social Services, Department of Welfare, or Health Department. Any of these agencies can tell you who in your state administers the program.

Medicaid may pay for nursing home services that are not covered by Medicare. This program is the most important third-party provider of funding for nursing home care in the United States today. Although it is sometimes administered through the Department of Welfare, many families who are not "welfare" recipients use this program to pay for needed quality care because of the enormous costs of nursing home care. Many people have strong feelings of discomfort about taking "welfare." It is important to remember that our taxes pay for these social programs and that when you are eligible for a program you are entitled by law to receive its benefits. The government has created these programs to help people.

Laws governing Medicaid programs vary with each state. Changes and reinterpretations of policy occur frequently. You may find it helpful to look into laws and regulations in your state before you need medical assistance. However, due to the frequent changes in regulations, agencies may be unable to give you specific answers about your status in advance of your application for assistance. You may also find it useful to consult a lawyer if you or the patient owns property or other assets.

Financial need for Medicaid and medical need for Medicaid are assessed separately.

Most of a person's income and assets must be spent on his care. When his income and assets are not enough to pay for his care in a nursing home, Medicaid makes up the difference. While the eligibility standards may seem unfair (and sometimes they unfairly impoverish a spouse), they are based on a legislative policy that tax money should be spent only on people who otherwise cannot receive care and should not be spent to allow individuals or families to save their own money.

The application for determination of financial eligibility for Medicaid is usually made by a competent family member for the individual needing nursing home placement. Make an appointment at the agency that processes applications. They will ask you to bring with you evidence of the patient's financial status. The documents required usually include his Social Security number, proof of income to the individual (Social Security benefit letters, pension benefit letters, etc.), bank account statements, insurance policies, and proof of any transfer of funds. Before going to the application appointment, ask about any other information you may need to bring.

You are entitled to a clear and courteous explanation of your eligibility status. In the event that you do not get an explanation you can accept or understand, ask to speak to the supervisor. As a last resort, each agency has an appeals system available to you. A social worker can be helpful to you in applying for Medicaid.

If Medicaid is granted, the actual payments to the nursing home will come from two sources. The first source is the individual patient's income from Social Security, pension plans, or insurance. The second is Medicaid, which pays the remainder of the cost.

Often the cost of nursing home care is borne first by one resource and then another. For example,

*Mrs. Campbell has Alzheimer's disease. She was cared for at home by her husband until she had a series of falls and*

*became unable to walk. Mr. Campbell took her to the hospital, where X-rays showed that she had broken her hip. The family decided that it was time for her to enter a nursing home. During the first 100 days her care was paid for by Medicare because she needed the skilled care of a nurse to help her hip heal. Then Mr. Campbell sold the stock his wife had inherited and was able to pay for her care for an additional six months with this money. At the end of that time he applied for Medicaid, which then paid for her care because she had no other source of income.*

Here are some of the questions that families often ask about Medicaid:

1. Are children or other relatives required to support their parents? In some states, sons or daughters are not legally considered responsible to support their parents. In others, part of a son's or daughter's income may be sought by the state for a parent's support. A person cannot be denied eligibility because a child refuses to pay, but the state can seek reimbursement through the courts.

2. Are spouses responsible for the support of the person in a nursing home? In all states the income of a spouse and jointly owned assets are considered if both are living together at the time of placement. However, in many states, the well spouse can no longer be held financially responsible after the ill spouse has been in a nursing home for a certain number of months (usually six months).

Often couples are living together on the retirement income of one of them, usually the husband. Since one's own income must be spent on one's nursing home care, when most of a couple's income belongs to the institutionalized partner, the well partner may be left without enough to live on. This can lead to serious hardship and is a major inequity in the law. A spouse, most often a wife, can be left with little or no income. For example.

*Mr. and Mrs. Blake live on his retirement income. Mrs. Blake has never worked. If Mr. Blake enters a nursing home, his retirement income must be spent on his nursing home costs. Mrs. Blake will be left with only her Social Security benefit as his dependent, which amounts to $210 a month. She will be unable to maintain their home or car.*

Nursing home placement can mean a significant loss of income to the spouse, particularly where the patient is the husband. The spouse may need to find additional funds for herself. If the spouse's income falls below a certain level and she is at least sixty-five years old, she can apply for Supplemental Security Income (SSI), a federal program for people without Social Security or other retirement income. This will raise her monthly income to (in 1981) approximately $265 a month. She may also qualify for food stamps and other social benefits. The total monthly income figure will be revised upward by the government periodically as the cost of living rises, but it usually remains at or near the poverty level.

3. Will I have to sell my house to be eligible? In most state, the home to which an institutionalized person could reasonably be expected to return or in which a spouse is living does *not* have to be sold. However, in most states the state can make a claim against the estate after the death of the spouse living in the house for reimbursement of nursing home costs. If the house was sold prior to placement, the capital must be spent on nursing home care.

4. Can I transfer the sick person's assets (land, stocks, property) out of his name to make him eligible for Medicaid? The laws governing the transfer of assets are being reassessed and revised by both the federal government and each state. If the patient has substantial assets, seek the help of a lawyer in advance of the time when he will need to enter a nursing home.

5. Can a nursing home reject a person on Medicaid?

Depending on state regulations, nursing homes can refuse to accept or keep a patient who entered a nursing home on Medicare or private funds and who eventually has to shift to Medicaid funds. Before entering a person in a nursing home, find out what the law in your state is regarding this and read the nursing home contract *carefully* to determine whether there is a clause in it that specifies that the patient will be kept if he must be supported by Medicaid.

In some areas the patient who is on Medicaid can be required to accept the first available bed even if it is in an unsuitable nursing home or one so far away that the family cannot visit. You need to know what to expect. A social worker may be able to help you.

### Establishing the Level of Medical Care

Once you have made a decision about how to pay for nursing home care, the family can proceed to the next step in the process, the establishment of medical need. If the person has been under close medical attention this step will probably be quie simple. Nursing homes require basic medical information about the patient and his treatments; many require a recent physical examination by his physician. Homes also require positive proof that the patient does not have tuberculosis, so the patient may need to have a new chest X-ray. If the person will be paying for his own care (or if the family is paying), this may be all that is necessary.

If the person will be supported by Medicare he must be certified as needing skilled care and he must meet Medicare criteria. If the person will be supported by Medicaid, the level of medical need must be established (skilled care, intermediate care, etc.). The terms for levels of care vary with different states, but they describe the amount of nursing care he will need.

After the doctor has examined the patient, he will fill out a standard form. This form will be sent to a review organization, who will decide what kind of nursing home care is most appropriate for the patient. A *level-of-care rating* (a definition of how much nursing care a person requires) will be assigned to the patient. Each level of care provides for different services to the patient. All states make a level-of-care determination when a person enters a nursing home. This level of care decides whether the patient is medically eligible for Medicare or Medicaid, at what level payment will be made, and what kind of home the person may enter.

A social worker or a nurse can help you with this process. If you have questions about the process in your state, ask your physician or the local Department of Social Services/ Department of Public Welfare.

Every nursing home has specific numbers of beds assigned at specific levels of care, but a given home may not have all levels of care. A person can only enter a home that has an available bed at the assigned level of care. With a few exceptions, a person may not occupy a bed designated at a more skilled level than his needs are determined to be.

At present all states require a periodic review of the patient's condition by a physician and a designated review agency. If a person gets better in a nursing home he may encounter a bureaucratic "catch 22." For example,

*Mr. Girard has Alzheimer's disease. He entered a nursing home because he had a broken hip. After about eight months, his hip had healed and the good care the staff gave him got him back on his feet. The review agency found that he no longer needed skilled nursing care and he was not eligible to remain in the skilled nursing facility or to continue to receive Medicaid payments at the skilled level. There was no bed available at the intermediate care level. His dementia had gotten worse and his family was unable to care for him at home. There was nowhere for him to go.*

Patients often get worse when they are moved from one nursing home to another, and beds at other levels of care are not always available, especially for people receiving Medicaid, so there may be no place for a person who gets better to go. Some states have passed laws addressing this dilemma. You need to know where you stand before the problem arises.

## Finding a Home or Facility

The third step in this process is finding a suitable home for your family member. This process will differ depending on whether the person goes directly from the hospital to a nursing home or directly from home to a nursing home. If the person goes directly from the hospital, there is usually a social worker on the hospital staff who will help you arrange the placement. Be sure to ask if there is such a staff person. A social worker will be able to help you establish financial and medical eligibility, and can provide you ith a list of nursing homes in your area. The social worker may be able to help with other steps in the total process as well, and can also help you with the painful feelings you may be having about the placement.

If the person is to go from home to a nursing home, you may be able to locate a social worker in the Department of Social Services, the Department of Welfare, your local Commission on Aging (if one of you is over sixty), or a family service agency, or even get a private social worker. The social worker will provide you ith a list of homes and help you with the eligibility process. Nursing homes are listed in the yellow pages of the phone directory; good homes may be known to other families in your community, or your doctor may recommend a good home.

When you have a list of possible homes, call to make an appointment to see the administrator and/or the director of nursing and to visit the home. There are some fundamental questions you might ask on the telephone before you visit the home. First, you will need to find out if the home has beds for the level-of-care rating to which the patient has been assigned. The home may have beds, but have a waiting list. You should go to see the home if it has a waiting list; if it is a good home you may wish to place the patient on the list. Second, you will need to find out if the home accepts the funding sources you are planning to use.

It is not always easy to find available beds in good homes, especially if the person is going to be receiving Medicaid. Medicaid programs pay nursing homes less than the home can charge people who are paying for their own care; therefore, many good homes will not accept more Medicaid patients than regulations require them to accept. In many areas there are not enough Medicaid beds. You may have no choice but to accept a home that does not meet all of your expectations.

When you visit the home you will need to observe and ask questions. When meeting with nursing home administrators you should feel free to ask questions about the home's accreditation, financial procedures, and quality of care.

Most qualified nursing homes participate in two voluntary standards programs. One is accreditation by the Long-Term Council of the Joint Commission on Accreditation of Hospitals. This is based on on-site surveys in which the facility's operations are evaluated in terms of substantial compliance with the commission's standards. The other is peer review, which helps improve the quality of care through systematic review of the facility by fellow members of the American Health Care Association's (AHCA) individual state affiliates. Since the AHCA approved this professional review system in 1971, more than half the states have formed their own peer review committees to better assure quality care.

When you meet with nursing home administrators, discuss financial arrangements in detail. Do not take anything for granted. If there are things you do not understand, don't hesitate to ask. All financial agreements should be in writing, and you should have a copy of the final arrangements. You may wish to cover the following areas before signing the papers:

1. Will the patient or resident receive a refund of advance payments if he leaves the facility?
2. How are cash and assets that have been entrusted to the home protected? Is a receipt given to the patient? Are withdrawals noted by signed receipt, so that you or the resident can keep track of his account?
3. Are the agreed date of admission and the degree of care to be furnished set forth in the written agreement?
4. Under what circumstances can the home discharge a person, and how much notice must they give you?
5. Will the home retain the person when his private funds are expended and he transfers his method of payment to Medicaid funding?
6. If there is potential for the person to improve (from an acute illness, for example), can he be transferred to a different level of care *within the same home*, so that he does not have to move?

If the staff is reluctant to answer your questions, this may be an indication of how you will be treated after placement.

We have included a checklist of questions that you may want to ask as you visit homes. These will help you evaluate the quality of care the home provides. You may want to take it along with you. There are three vital questions:

1. Does the home have a current license from the state?
2. Does the administrator have a current license from the state?
3. Does the home meet or exceed state fire regulations? It is difficult to evacuate frail elderly people in case of fire. Sprinkler systems and fire doors are important.

If the above questions cannot be answered yes, do not use the home.

4. If Medicare and/or Medicaid is needed, is the home certified to accept it? (If you will pay from another source initially and then switch to Medicaid, you need to know whether the home will keep the patient.)
5. Is the home accredited by the Long-Term Care Council of the Joint Commission on Accreditation of Hospitals?
6. Has the home been reviewed by your state health care or nursing home association's peer review committee?
7. Do you clearly understand what costs are included in the basic charge and what costs, such as laundry, medications, haircuts, incontinence pads, special nursing procedures, etc., are extra?
8. Is there a low staff turnover? Ask the administrator. Staff of good nursing homes recommend this as an excellent clue to the level of staff satisfaction.
9. Does the staff seem happy and friendly? Happy personnel indicate a well-run institution. Also, contented people are less likely to take out their personal frustrations on the residents.
10. Is the home, including nonpatient areas, such as kitchens, clean? It may be impossible to keep it spotless, but the area should seem clean.
11. Are bathrooms and other areas equipped with grab bars, hand rails, no-skid floors, and other devices for patient safety?
12. What arrangements does the home have for transporting acutely ill people to the hospital? How are medical problems handled?
13. States set standards for safety and medical care. Has the home met these?
14. Has the staff been trained to notice and evaluate changes in mental functioning?

15. Are the aides given training on how to care for people with dementing illnesses? The staff need to know how to manage catastrophic reactions, suspiciousness, wandering, etc. (If they are not given this training, do they welcome the information you offer them?)

16. Are provisions made for people who wander or who become agitated? You may see people in restraints, but this should not be the usual way to manage behavior. Use of restraints over prolonged periods is rarely necessary. Other nursing management techniques will handle most problems. Many states have laws governing the use of restraints (see Appendix 5). Wanderers need to be protected from open doors and stairs.

17. Is the home convenient for you to visit? Can the resident's private physician visit?

18. Does the home have long visiting hours? If visiting is restricted to only a few hours, one wonders what goes on when no family members are around. May children visit?

19. Is the home pleasant to be in, and well lighted, the staff cheerful, the furniture comfortable, residents' personal possessions in sight in their rooms? Pleasant surroundings and kind, patient staff are very important to a confused person. You also need to feel comfortable when you come to visit.

20. Do you think the patient will feel comfortable here? There are "homey" homes that may smell a little and have worn furniture but that may seem more like home to some people, while other people will feel more comfortable in a newer facility.

21. Are individual diets available? Is the food wholesome, attractive, and suitable for elderly people?

22. Are meals adequate? Are residents who need help receiving it at mealtime? Are snacks available? Volunteers may be used to help people at mealtimes.

23. Are people with swallowing problems closely supervised? Long-term use of nasogastric (NG) tubes or other devices that circumvent voluntary eating are not recommended if good nursing management will enable a person to eat.

24. How are the incontinent patients manated? Nursing management of incontinent people is usually superior to continuous use of catheters.

25. Is bowel and bladder retraining available for residents who can benefit from it?

26. Are programs available to keep residents alert and involved within the limits of their abilities?

27. Is supervised daily exercise provided? Even wheelchair and bed patients need exercise, and those who can walk should be doing so. Exercise may reduce the restlessness of people with dementing illnesses.

28. Are there creative and effective planned social activities? A TV room is not enough. Nursing home residents need structured programs such as music programs, recreation groups, and outings to keep them involved in interpersonal activities at the level of their abilities.

29. Are physical therapy, speech therapy, and occupational or recreational therapy available to residents who need it?

30. Do clergy visit regularly and can residents attend religious services?

31. Do residents wear their own clothes, have locked private storage space, have privacy for letters and phone calls? Can they have privacy with visitors, and is private space provided for visits from a spouse?

32. Does the home have a social worker? A social worker can help you with many of the problems and adjustments that may arise.

33. Is there a resident council that can take problems and

complaints to the administrator? Where can you take complaints?
34. Some states have established a Patient's Bill of Rights. Is such a bill of rights available in your state and does the home comply with it? (A sample Patient Bill of Rights is included in Appendix 5.)

Ideally you should be able to answer yes to many of these questions. In reality, such quality care is expensive and hard to find. If the person is difficult to manage or if you must rely on Medicaid funding, you may not be able to find an ideal home. Use these questions as a guide to help you decide which things are most important and which ones you are willing to compromise on.

## Moving to the Nursing Home

Once a nursing home has been found and financial arrangements have been made, the next step is the actual transfer to the home. We have discussed helping the impaired person move on p. 66. Many of the same things are important when a person moves to a nursing home.

Tell the person where he is going if you think there is any chance he will understand. Take familiar items that he is fond of with him (pictures, mementos, an afghan or radio). If possible, he should help select these. Even a person who is upset or severely impaired needs to feel that this is his life and he is still important. You may have to close your ears to his accusations if he blames you for this move. However, if he repeatedly becomes upset when the home is mentioned, we do not feel it is helpful to keep mentioning it. You may need to go on matter-of-factly with arrangements. Try to avoid dishonest explanations such as "we are going for a ride" or "you are going for a visit." This can make the person's subsequent adjustment in the nursing home more difficult.

You may not find a nursing home you really like or you may feel that the staff is not giving the patient the kind of care he should receive. However, you may not have any alternative but to leave the person in that home. The director of an excellent home suggests that you avoid complaints and do all that you can to establish a friendly relationship with the staff. This may mean a compromise on your part, but may well encourage their cooperation. Offer them information about dementia.

If you are moving the person from a hospital to the nursing home, you may have little or no time to search for a good home and to plan an orderly transition. You may be exhausted by all that must be done in a few hours or days. If this happens, at least try to go with the person to the home and to have some familiar things waiting there for him.

## Adjusting to a New Life

The change to living in a nursing home means major adjustments for the impaired person. Making these adjustments takes time and energy for staff, residents, and family, and it can be a painful process. Remember that the move to a nursing home need not mean the end of family relationships. Your relative can continue to be a part of the family even though he has moved into a setting that better meets his needs. There are some practical suggestions for things that you can do to make the adjustment to the new home easier. However, we know that the difficult part of the adjustment is the feelings you and your relative may have about it.

You can help your relative orient himself in his new home. While you are visiting, explain again why he is here (for example, say, ''You are too sick to stay at home'') and what the daily routines of the home are (making a schedule for him if he can read it). Help him find the bathroom, dining room, TV, and phone. Help him find his things in his closet. Think of a way to identify the door of his room as his. Decorate his room with things that are his.

Tell him exactly when you will visit next and write this down for him so he can use it to remind himself. Try to continue to involve him in family outings. If he is not acutely ill, take him for rides, shopping, home for dinner or overnight, or to church. Even if he resists going back he may eventually come to accept this routine and he will benefit from the knowledge that he is still part of the family. Occasionally it continues to be difficult to get the person to return. In this instance it is better to visit him at the home.

Help him to remain a part of special family events such as birthdays and holidays. Even if he is depressed or confused he usually should still be informed of sad events. It is rarely a ''kindness'' not to tell a person about a death, unless there is an urgent medical reason not to tell him. If you do not tell him of a death he may wonder why this person has abandoned him and no longer visits. If he does not remember that someone has died, accept this. His memory impairment may make it impossible for him to remember what you tell him. We do not feel that repeating such information is necessary if the person is unable to remember and does not ask.

Telephone calls between visits help a forgetful person keep in touch and remind him that he is not forgotten. Don't expect him to be able to remember to call you.

Take an old photograph album, an old dress from the attic, or some other item that may trigger memories of the past and urge the person to talk about things he remembers from long ago. If he always tells you the same story, accept this. It is your listening to him that communicates that you still care about him.

Talk about the family, the neighbors, gossip. Even if the person is not fully aware of the issues, he can enjoy the act of listening and talking. Being together is important to both of you. Confused people may not be interested in some topics, such as current events. If the person seems restless, do not insist on bringing him up to date on information.

Be sympathetic about his complaints. Listening to the things he complains about tells him that you care about him. He may make the same complaint over and over because he forgets that he told you. Listen anyway; it is your empathy he needs. Investigate his complaint thoughtfully, however, before you complain to the staff or act on it. Remember that his perception of things may not be accurate.

Sing old, familiar songs. Don't be surprised if other residents drift by to listen or participate. Music is a wonderful way to share. Nobody will remember if your singing isn't very good. Take tape recordings of the family or the children.

Avoid too much excitement. Your arrival, news, and conversation may overexcite the impaired person and could precipitate a catastrophic reaction.

Do things that show that you are interested in his new home. Walk around it together, read the bulletin board to him, talk to his roommate or other residents and staff. Remind him to smell the flowers and see the birds when you walk around outside.

Help him care for himself. Eat a meal together, do his hair, rub his back, hold hands, help him get some exercise. Bring a treat that you can eat together while you are there. Avoid bringing food the staff must store. If the person has difficulty eating, you may want to come at mealtimes and help feed him. If other confused or upset residents interrupt your visit, you may be able to tell them gently but clearly not to talk with you now. If necessary, ask if there is a more private place for you to visit.

If he enjoys it and if it does not precipitate a catastrophic reaction, take along children (one at a time) or a pet (ask the staff in advance). Seeing the people in a home is usually helpful for children. You can prepare the child by talking about the things he might see such as catheters or intravenous tubes and explaining that they help such people maintain their bodily functions.

Sometimes a person is so ill that he cannot talk, cannot recognize you or respond to you. It is hard to know what to say to such a person. Try holding hands, rubbing the person's back, or singing. One minister said this about his visits:

> *"I've grown in these visits. I am so used to doing, doing, doing and there is nothing I can do for these people. I've learned to just sit, to just share being and not to feel I have to do or talk or entertain."*

Sharing family life and loving a person who is in an institution and who is in the late stages of a dementing illness are not easy, but perhaps you will find your own meaning in doing so, as this man has.

You also will have changes in your life when a family member has moved to a nursing home. If the person lived with you, and especially when he is your spouse, the adjustment may be difficult. You may be tired from the efforts of arranging for placement and, on top of your fatigue, you may also feel sad at the changes that have happened. The move to a nursing home may intensify your feelings of grief and loss. At the same time you may wish that you could somehow have kept the person at home, and you may feel guilty that this was not possible. You may have mixed feelings of relief and sorrow, guilt and anger. It *is* a relief not to have to carry the burden of care, to be able to sleep or read uninterrupted. Still, you probably with things were different and that you could have continued to care for this person yourself.

Families often tell us that in the first few days they feel lost. Without the usual demands of caring for a sick person, they cannot decide what to do with themselves. At first you may not be able to sleep through the night or relax enough to watch television.

The trips to the nursing home may be tiring, especially if

the home is some distance from where you live. The visits may be depressing. Sometimes confused people are temporarily worse until they adjust to a new setting, and this can upset you. Sometimes, too, the other people in the home are depressing to see.

Nursing home staff are geared to provide care for many people and you may not feel that your loved one is getting the individual care that you would like. Other things about the home or the staff may upset you. It's not unusual for you to feel angry with nursing home staff from time to time. If you are upset with the home or the staff you have a right to discuss your concerns with them, to be given answers, and not to jeopardize the patient's care or status in the home by doing this. No home should be able to discharge a resident because you have raised questions about his care.

If there is a social worker in the home, she may help you work out your concerns. If there is not, discuss your concerns in a calm, matter-of-fact way with the administrator or the director of nurses.

Sometimes serious problems about patient care do arise.

*Mr. Rosen says, "My father has Alzheimer's disease and we had to put him in a nursing home. He got terribly sick and was transferred to a hospital, where they said his condition was made worse because he was dehydrated. Apparently the home failed to give him enough fluid. I feel like I am guilty of not checking up on this and I feel like I can't send him back to a home that neglects him."*

As you know, people with dementing illnesses can be difficult to care for, especially in the late stages of the disease. If Mr. Rosen complains to the nursing home staff he may only make them angry; if he tries to move his father to another home, he may find there are no other homes that are any better or that will accept a person with Alzheimer's disease or who is receiving Medicaid.

The dilemma you, Mr. Rosen, and many other families fact lies not so much with one home but with national policy, value systems, federal training budgets, and so forth. These things are gradually changing through the efforts of organizations such as ADRDA. We hope that you will not encounter dilemmas like this. If you do, try talking over your concerns honestly but calmly with the administrator, nursing director, or social worker and offer her the information you have about the care of people with dementing illnesses.

Often things are better after placement, especially when they have been difficult at home. With other people responsible for daily care, you and the patient can relax and enjoy each other. Since you are not always tired, and can get away from the person's irritating behaviors, you may be able to relax and enjoy your relationship for the first time.

If other family members do not visit, it may be because they find it very hard to face visiting in a nursing home, don't know what to talk about, and so don't come. If someone in your family reacts this way, try to understand that this may be their way of grieving and you may not be able to change them.

Sometimes family members spend many hours at the nursing home, helping with the patient. Only you can decide how much time you should spend visiting. Ask yourself in part of your reason for being there has to do with your loneliness and your grief and might it be better if you spent less time there so the resident can make his adjustment to his new home.

Time does pass, and gradually the acute phase of adjustment also passes. As time goes on you will settle into a routine of visits. It is natural for you gradually to build a life apart from the person who has changed so much.

## Sexual Issues in Nursing Homes

Sometimes confused residents in nursing homes undress themselves in public, masturbate, or make advances to staff or other residents. The sexual needs and behaviors of residents in nursing homes have recently become a controversial issue. Sexual behavior in a nursing home differs in significant ways from such behaviors at home: it no longer is a private matter, but in one way or another has an impact on staff, other residents, and the families of residents; and it raises the ethical issue of whether a person who is impaired can or should retain the right to make sexual decisions for himself.

While our culture seems to be saturated with talk about sex, it is the sexuality of the young and beautiful that is being discussed. Most of us are uncomfortable considering the sexuality of the old, the unattractive, the handicapped, or the demented. Nursing home staff also often feel uncomfortable.

If the nursing home staff reports inappropriate behavior to you, remember that much of the behavior that at first seems sexual is really behavior of disorientation and confusion. You and the nursing home staff can work together to help the person know where he is, when he can use the toilet, and where he can undress. Often all that is needed is to say "It isn't time to go to bed yet. We'll put your pajamas on later." Distractions, such as offering a glass of juice, are helpful.

Confused persons may become close friends with another resident, often without a sexual relationship. Friendship is a universal need that does not stop when one becomes demented. Occasionally one hears stories about people getting in bed with other residents in a nursing home. This is not hard to understand when we consider that most of us have shared a bed with someone for many years and have enjoyed the closeness this sharing brings. The confused person may not realize where he is or whom he is with. He may not realize that he is not in his own bed. He may feel that he is with his spouse. Remember that nursing homes can be lonely places where there is not much opportunity for being held and loved. How you respond to such an incident depends on your attitudes and values and on the response of the nursing home.

Some nursing home residents masturbate. The staff usually ignores such behavior, which is usually done in the person's room. If it occurs in public the person should be quietly returned to his room.

Some men make overtures to the nursing home staff. The irony of this is that many men have always enjoyed flirting with the ladies without offending anyone. When the staff matter-of-factly and kindly sets limits, this behavior seldom becomes a problem.

## STATE MENTAL HOSPITALS

Occasionally a person with a dementing illness exhibits behaviors that are so difficult to manage that no nursing home will accept them. Such people may be placed in the geriatric unit of the state mental hospital. In some cases skilled medical and nursing management can reduce difficult behaviors and present state hospital placement. A consultation with a geriatric psychiatrist should be sought to attempt to avoid placement.

Just as there are some parents who neglect their children, occasionally there are families who do not want to care for an aging member. Or once in a while a family will want to place a person in the state hospital to avoid having to pay for nursing home care. Usually the state will require that the person's income and assets be spent on his care under the same regulations that govern Medicaid in nursing homes.

State hospitals have been mandated by the legislature to reduce their geriatric patient populations and so are reluctant to accept new patients. Some areas have programs whose responsibility it is to prevent placement in state hospitals if possible by mobilizing other resources. These are staffed by physicians, nurses, or social workers who have expertise in helping you avoid state hospitalization. Because of this policy of deinstitutionalization and because of funding cuts, some state hospitals will not accept dementia patients, and it can be difficult to find a place for a problem patient. You may need the help of a physician, social worker, clergyman, or even your congressman.

State mental hospitals have a bad reputation. Some do provide good care. Most are doing the best they can within their limitations. Others have earned their bad reputation. You will want to learn how your hospital is regarded by local physicians.

If a person does enter a state hospital, you can continue to visit and maintain family ties as you would if he were in a nursing home.

# 17

## BRAIN DISORDERS AND THE CAUSES OF DEMENTIA

SOMETIMES the brain does not work as it should. Such problems may be called retardation, dyslexia, dementia, or psychosis. They may be caused by an injury to the brain, a genetic condition, chemicals in the environment which are damaging the brain, or many other things. In this chapter we will explain how dementia differs from other problems of the brain and describe some of the most common causes of dementia.

## DEMENTIA

Doctors and scientists group the different things that can go wrong with the brain by their symptoms. Just as fever, coughing, vomiting, and dizziness are symptoms of several different diseases, memory loss, confusion, personality change, and problems with speaking are also symptoms of several diseases.

*Dementia* is the medical term for a group of symptoms. It describes a global decline in intellectual ability sufficiently severe to interfere with a person's daily functioning which occurs in a person who is awake and alert (not drowsy, intoxicated, or unable to pay attention). This decline in intellectual functioning means a loss of several kinds of mental processes that may include mathematical ability, vocabulary, abstract thinking, judgment, speaking, or coordination. It may include changes in personality. "Not feeling quite as sharp as you used to" does not mean that one is developing a dementia. The person's ability must decline from what was normal for him. This is different from mental retardation, in which a person has been impaired since infancy.

These symptoms of dementia can be caused by many diseases. Some of the diseases are treatable; some are not. In some, the dementia can be stopped; in some it can be reversed; in others the primary condition cannot be changed. Some of these diseases are rare. Other diseases are not rare, but the people who have them do not usually become demented. Do not assume that a dementia is the inevitable result of having these diseases. A *partial* list of the conditions that can cause dementia follows:

Metabolic disorders
  Thyroid, parathyroid, or adrenal gland dysfunction
  Liver or kidney dysfunction
  Certain vitamin deficiencies, such as vitamin B-12 deficiency
Structural problems of the brain
  Normal pressure hydrocephalus (abnormal flow of spinal fluid)
  Brain tumors
  Subdural hematoma (bleeding beneath the skull which results in collections of blood which press on the brain)
  Trauma (injuries to the brain)

    Hypoxia and anoxia (insufficient oxygen)
Infections
    Tuberculosis
    Syphilis
    Fungal, bacterial, and viral infections of the brain, such as meningitis or encephalitis
Toxins (poisons)
    Carbon monoxide
    Drugs
    Metal poisoning
    Alcohol (Scientists disagree about whether alcohol can cause dementia.)
Degenerative diseases (causes generally unknown)
    Alzheimer's disease
    Friedreich's ataxia
    Huntington's disease
    Parkinson's disease
    Pick's disease
    Progressive supranuclear palsy
    Wilson's disease
Vascular (blood vessel) disease
    Stroke or multi-infarct disease
Autoimmune diseases
    Temporal arthritis
    Lupus erythematosus
Psychiatric diseases
    Depression
    Schizophrenia
Multiple sclerosis

Korsakoff's syndrome causes an impairment only in memory and not in other mental functions. It looks like a dementing illness but, because it affects only one area of mental function, it is not a true dementia.

Most research indicates that about 50 percent of the cases

of dementia are caused by Alzheimer's disease, 20 percent are caused by multi-infarct disease, and 20 percent are caused by a combination of Alzheimer's disease and multi-infarct disease. About 10 percent of the cases of dementia are caused by one or another of all the remaining conditions.

## Alzheimer's Disease

Alzheimer's disease was first described by a German physician. Alois Alzheimer, in 1907 and the condition was named for him. The disease Alzheimer originally described occurred in a woman in her fifties and was called *presenile dementia*. Neurologists now agree that the dementia that occurs in the elderly is the same as or similar to the presenile condition. It is usually called senile dementia of the Alzheimer's type *(SDAT)*.

The symptoms of the disease usually are a gradual though sometimes imperceptible decline in many areas of intellectual abilities and an accompanying physical decline. Early in the illness only memory may be noticeably impaired. The person is more than a little forgetful. She may have difficulty learning new skills or difficulty with tasks that require abstract reasoning or calculation, such as math. She may have trouble on the job or she may not enjoy reading as much as she used to. Her personality may change or she may become depressed.

Later, impairment in both language and motor abilities are seen. At first the person will be unable to find the right word for things or will use the wrong word, but she will gradually become unable to express herself. She will also have increasing trouble understanding explanations. She may give up reading or stop watching television. She may have increasing difficulty doing tasks that once were easy for her. Her handwriting may change or she may walk with a stoop or shuffle or become clumsy. She may get lost easily, forget that she has turned on the stove, misunderstand what is going on, show poor judgment. She may have changes in her personality or uncharacteristic outbursts of anger. She will be unable to plan responsibly for herself. Families often do not notice the beginnings of language and motor problems, but as the disease progresses all of these symptoms will become apparent.

Late in the illness the person becomes severely impaired, incontinent, and unable to walk or may fall frequently. She may be unable to say more than one or two words, and may recognize no one or only one or two people. She will need nursing care from you or from professionals. She will be physically disabled as well as intellectually impaired.

Alzheimer's disease usually leads to death in about seven to ten years, but it can progress more quickly (three to four years) or more slowly (as much as fifteen years).

Under a microscope, changes can be seen in the structure of the brain of a person who suffered from Alzheimer's disease. These include abnormally large numbers of structures called neuritic plaques and neurofibrillary tangles (see Chapter 18). This is clearly an injury to the brain itself. A diagnosis of Alzheimer's disease can be made on the basis of the type of symptoms, the way the symptoms progress over time, the absence of any other cause for the condition, and a compatible CAT scan. However, a final diagnosis of Alzheimer's disease rests on the presence of these specific abnormal structures (neuritic plaques and neurofibrillary tangles) in the brain tissue. A brain biopsy is the only way of making this determination. The biopsy is done by removing a piece of skull bone and taking out a small piece of brain tissue. The removal of this small amount of tissue has no effect on mental function. Brain biopsies are not routinely done at present because no treatment is available even if a diagnosis is made. This may change as research in dementia progresses.

## Multi-Infarct Dementia

In the past, dementing illnesses of old age were thought to be caused by *hardening of the arteries* of the brain. We now know that this is not the case. In multi-infarct dementia, repeated strokes within the brain destroy small areas of the brain. The cumulative effect of this damage leads to a dementia.

Multi-infarct dementias affect several functions, such as memory, coordination, or speech, but the symptoms differ somewhat depending on what areas of the brain are being damaged.

Multi-infarct dementias generally progress in a step-like way. You may be able to look back and recall that the person was worse after a specific time (instead of the gradual, imperceptible decline in Alzheimer's disease). Then she may not seem to get worse for a period, or she may even appear to get a little better. Some multi-infarct dementias progress as time passes; others may not get any worse for years. Somemulti-infarct dementias may be stopped by preventing further strokes; in others the progression cannot be stopped.

Some people may have both Alzheimer's disease and multi-infarct disease.

## Depression

Depression is a treatable cause of dementia. In a study of patients seen at The Johns Hopkins Hospital, about one-quarter of those who had symptoms of dementia were depressed. Eighty-two percent of these got better when the patient received treatment for the depression. That depression can cause dementia has been widely accepted only recently and occasionally a physician may not recognize dementia caused by depression. However, the symptoms of the depression are usually easily recognizable.

Whenever a person with a memory problem is depressed, she should be evaluated to determine whether the depression is the cause of her dementia or vice versa. Her depression should be treated whether or not she has an irreversible dementia. Do not allow a physician to dismiss depression. However, keep in mind that the person's depression may improve but not his memory problems.

## OTHER BRAIN DISORDERS

There are several other mental conditions that are not dementias.

### Delirium

The term *delirium* describes another *set of symptoms* that can have various causes. Delirium is often confused with dementia. Like the demented patient, the delirious patient may be forgetful or disoriented. Unlike a demented person, *the delirious person shows a reduced level of consciousness*. She may have a reduced ability to shift attention, focus attention, or sustain attention. Other symptoms of delirium may include misinterpretation of reality, false ideas, or hallucinations; incoherent speech; either sleepiness in the daytime or akefulness at night; and increased or decreased physical (motor) activity. Symptoms of delirium often develop over a few hours or days. They tend to vary through the day.

Older people who do not have dementing illnesses may show symptoms—often intermittent—of impaired alertness, confusion, or memory problems. This may be a delirium caused by some other illness or medication. Such a delirium should be regarded as a symptom, and the causative disease should be identified and treated, if possible.

People with dementing illnesses are vulnerable to developing a delirium in addition to their dementia. You may observe a sudden worsening in a person who also has other problems, such as constipation, the flu, an infection, or even a slight cold. It is important to treat any such problem, because even very minor problems can seriously affect a person with a dementing illness.

## Senility, Chronic Organic Brain Syndrome, Acute or Reversible Organic Brain Syndromes

The word *senile* merely means "old." Thus, senility does not describe a disease and is considered by many people to be derogatory or prejudicial.

*Chronic organic brain syndrome* and *acute or reversible organic brain syndromes* are terms used by some to refer to those dementias that could not be treated (chronic) and to deliriums that respond to treatment (acute), respectively. These terms are no longer used because they are not specific and because they include implications of prognosis. We hope that in time there will be no "chronic" brain symdromes.

### TIA

TIA stands for transient ischemic attack. This is a temporary impairment due to an insufficient supply of blood to part of the brain. The person may be unable to speak, or may have slurred speech. She may be weak or paralyzed, dizzy or nauseated. These symptoms usually last only a few minutes or hours before the person recovers. This is in contrast to a stroke which may have the same symptoms but after which some deficit remains. very small deficits may not be noticeable. TIAs should be regarded as warnings of stroke and should be reported to your doctor.

### Localized Brain Injuries

Damage can happen to the brain or head which temporarily or permanently affects either small or greater parts of the brain. This can be caused by brain tumors, strokes, or head injuries. Unlike dementia, such injuries may not be global, although they may affect more than one mental function. The symptoms can tell a neurologist just where the damage is. This is called a focal (localized) brain lesion (injury). When the damage is widespread the symptoms may be those of dementia.

Major *stroke,* which causes such things as sudden paralysis of one side of the body, drooping of one side of the face, or speech problems, is an injury to part of the brain. Strokes can be caused by a blood clot blocking vessels in the brain or by a blood vessel bursting and causing bleeding in the brain. Often the brain cells are injured or imparied by swelling but can recover when the swelling goes down. It may be that other parts of the brain can gradually learn to do the jobs of damaged sections of the brain. People who have had a stroke may get better. Rehabilitation training is important for people who have had a stroke. The chance of having another stroke can be reduced by good medical management.

## Head Injuries

Head injuries can destroy brain tissue directly or can cause bleeding within the brain. Sometimes blood collects between the skull and the brain, forming a pool of blood. This puts pressure on the brain cells and damages them. It is called a *subdural hematoma.* Even mild falls can cause such bleeding.

People with dementing diseases are vulnerable to falls and may not be able to tell you about them. If you suspect that a person has banged her head, she should be seen promptly by a doctor because treatment can prevent permanent damage. The bleeding beneath the skull may not occur in the same place as the head was hit.

# 18

## RESEARCH IN DEMENTIA

WE HAVE REACHED an exciting point in research into dementia. Not too long ago, most people assumed that dementia was the natural result of aging and only a few pioneers were interested in studying it. In the last ten years that has changed. It is now known that:

1. dementia is not the natural result of aging,
2. it is caused by specific, identifiable diseases,
3. diagnosis is important to identify treatable conditions,
4. a proper evaluation is important in the management of contributing diseases that at present are not curable.

Today an increasing amount of research is forcusing on the dementing illnesses. With new tools for study we can get a much clearer look at what goes on in the brain. Because of better public understanding, there is a growing demand for solutions. These factors acting together have attracted talented men and women to the study of dementia and we hope they will encourage allocation of more research money.

Much of the current research is supported by the National Institute of Neurological and Communicative Disorders and Stroke (NINCDS), the National Institute of Mental Health (NIMH), and the National Institute on Aging (NIA); NIA has published a summary of current research (see Appendix 1).

## UNDERSTANDING RESEARCH

Understanding and interpreting *what* the research data mean is sometimes difficult for scientists and families alike. Here are some things you need to know about research to help you understand what you read.

It is essential that studies carefully define their terms. For example, some researchers have studied people with "organic brain syndrome." Data from such a study can be misleading because we do not know whether the people had Alzheimer's disease or other illnesses.

There is a difference between a relationship between two things and proof that one thing causes the other. We may find both A and B in the brains of dementia patients, but this does not mean that A caused B. A and B might both have been caused by an unknown factor, C.

It is essential that studies eliminate the influence of other factors. Sometimes when a new technique or drug is tried, the patient gets better. The hopes of the doctor, the patient, and the family, the additional attention, or some other factor may affect his improvement. This is called the placebo effect and it is quite common. Good studies of drugs, for example, are carefully designed to eliminate the possibility that other factors cause improvement. When you hear that several people get better on a certain drug, it may be because either they did not have the same illness or the placebo effect caused temporary improvement.

It is important to know what studies of laboratory animals mean. Researchers who work with animals take into account in which ways the animals' reactions are similar to human reactions and in which ways they are not. Giving enormous doses of a chemical to an animal with a short life span magnifies the chances of seeing a relationship between the chemical and a disease, if one exists.

Epidemiology is the study of the distribution of diseases in large groups of people. The epidemiology of dementing illnesses may eventually show scientists a link between a dementing illness and something else as yet unknown—for example, a hereditary factor, diet in childhood, or use of a medicine many years ago. If you have participated in research programs, you may have been asked many questions that don't seem in any way related to your problem, but which give researchers important epidemiologic information.

The increased public awareness of Alzheimer's disease has been accompanied by increased advertising of "cures." Some of these are expensive, dangerous, ineffective, or unfairly raise hopes. The Alzheimer's Disease and Related Disorders Association can tell you which treatments are generally believed by doctors to be of no value.

Following is a summary of some of the research you may have read or heard about.

## Research in Multi-Infarct Dementia and Stroke

Scientists are seeking to determine what effects hypertension, obesity, diet, smoking, heart disease, and other factors have on a person's vulnerability to stroke or multi-infarct disease. They are studying which areas of the brain are most likely to be damaged and the changes in brain chemistry that take place after a stroke. They are looking at how, when, and to what extent rehabilitative training helps a person. They are examining the effect of drugs on preventing stoke, on dilating blood vessels, on increasing the oxygen supply to the brain, and on preventing clotting.

## Research in Alzheimer's Disease

### Neurotransmitters

Researchers have discovered that chemicals in the brain called *neuro-transmitters* are necessary for messages to pass from one nerve cell to the next. They have learned that in some diseases there is less than the normal amount of a certain neurotransmitter. For example, a patient with Parkinson's disease can take L-Dopa, which increases the amount of the deficient neurotransmitter dopamine and alleviates the symptoms.

Scientists know that people with Alzheimer's disease have a deficiency of the enzyme *choline acetyltransferase,* which is necessary to produce the neurotransmitter *acetylcholine.* Thus, acetylcholine is presumed deficient in the brain of people with Alzheimer's disease. Research is under way to find a way to increase the amount of acetylcholine in the brain or to find a drug that mimics it. Other neurotransmitters, such as somatostatin, may also be deficient.

Researchers have recently learned that a small area of the brain, the Nucleus Basalis of Meynert, shows cell loss in patients with Alzheimer's disease. Moreover, it now appears that this area is the site from which the brain's acetylcholine originates. It may be that plaques and tangles are remaining fragments of the cells which contained acetylcholine.

### Structural Brain Changes

It has long been known that there are microscopic changes in the brain of people with Alzheimer's disease called neuritic senile plaques and neurofibrillary tangles. These are found in much smaller quantities in the brain of normal older people. Scientists are analyzing their structure and chemistry for clues to their formation and what their role in the disease may be.

## Nutrition

Lecithin and choline, substances occurring in many foods, are known to be used by the body to make acetylcholine. Studies have been done in which lecithin has been given to groups of demented people. The results are disappointing but many issues need to be looked at more closely. More needs to be known about why acetylcholine appears to be in short supply in some brains. Families often try giving people lecithin bought from a health food store, but there is no evidence that this can improve memory, mood, or behavior.

## Metals

Aluminum has been found in larger than expected amounts in the brains of some people with Alzheimer's disease. Other metals, such as manganese, are known to be associated with other forms of dementia. It now seems most likely that the presence of aluminum is a result of whatever is causing the dementia rather than itself a cause of the dementia. People sometimes wonder if they should stop taking antacids or cooking with aluminum pans or using deodorants (all sources of aluminum.) There is no evidence that their use is a cause of dementia. Studies of people who have been exposed to much larger amounts of aluminum indicate that exposure does not lead to dementia. Some studies of drugs that assist in the elimination of aluminum from the body are being conducted.

## Viruses

Some tentative research led scientists to suspect that a viral disease could be causing Alzheimer's disease. you may read about Creutzfeldt-Jacob disease or Kuru. Both of these rare diseases have been studied because they appear to be transmitted by a viruslike agent. There is no direct evidence at present to support the hypothesis that Alzheimer's disease is caused by a slow virus, but research is actively going on to determine this.

## Drugs

Researchers are studying many compounds for the effects on memory. From time to time various drugs are proposed to treat people who have dementing illnesses. So far, however, none of them has been found to be effective when it is carefully tested in the laboratory, in spite of initial reports of people who improved. New drugs continue to be tested. You may hear about many of them. Some of these will lead to new treatments. Others will not be used after careful studies indicate that they are not effective.

## Immunological Defects

The immune system is the body's defense against infection. Studies of some of the proteins that the body uses to fight infection show abnormal levels in patients with Alzheimer's disease.

Scientists suspect that sometimes the body's defense system, which is designed to attack outside cells such as disease organisms, goes awry and attacks cells in the body. One theory is that this is what is happening in Alzheimer's disease. Numerous studies are being done approaching the problem fromt his angle.

## Neuropsychology

Neuropsychology is the study of the relationship between brain structure and behavior. Neuropsychologists are developing more sophisticated ways to diagnose Alzheimer's disease and to determine exactly which parts of the brain are being affected.

## Other Approaches

Other researchers are studying blood flow to the brain, genetic background, and the histories of demented patients. Perhaps from such studies some clue will emerge that will point to a cause of the disease. So far no such clues have been conclusive. One new and exciting tool is positron emission transaxial tomography (PETT), which will enable scientists to see just which parts of the brain are active when the brain does specific things. Comparing the results of normal and sick people should give clues to what is not working in the brains of people with dementing illnesses.

## THE ROLE OF HEREDITY

Families often ask if this disease is inherited or if later generations are likely to get Alzheimer's disease. An adult's chances of developing Alzheimer's disease are about 1 or 2 in 100 at age sixty-five but the odds increase fourfold if a close relative has the disease. These data, plus evidence that the disease may be related to other diseases such as Down's syndrome (Mongolism) known to be caused by defects in chromosomes, lead investigators to suspect that there may be a genetic factor in Alzheimer's disease. A genetic factor may mean a person has inherited a *tendency* to be more vulnerable to the disease but not that he will necessarily develop the disease.

Some investigators believe that women are more prone to Alzheimer's disease than men, but that men are more prone to multi-infarct dementia. This may be simply because men are more likely to develop vascular disease, while women tend to live longer and the incidence of Alzheimer's disease increases with age. Scientists are looking for clues to whether this is so.

## KEEPING ACTIVE

People often wonder if keeping mentally alert and involved or maintaining physical exercise will prevent a person from developing a dementing illness. As far as is known, neither physical exercise nor keeping mentally active will prevent or alter the course of Alzheimer's disease. Activity will help to maintain general health and improve the quality of life. Some studies that did not differentiate among causes of dementia have produced misleading results about the effect of activity on dementia. Sometimes people seem to develop a dementia after they retire. Upon close examination, however, it usually appears that the early stages of a dementia were developing before the person retired and that this early, unidentified dementia may have been a factor in the person's decision to retire.

## THE EFFECT OF ACUTE ILLNESS ON DEMENTIA

Sometimes people appear to develop a dementia after a serious illness, hospitalization, or surgery. Again, as far as is known, these things do not affect or alter the course of Alzheimer's dementia. Upon close examination it often is clear that the dementing illness had begun before the person had surgery or developed another disease. The stress of the acute illness and the tendency of people with a dementia to develop a delirium make the person worse, so his dementia is noticeable for the first time. Then the brain impairment will make it more difficult for him to adjust after his illness and he will *seem* more demented.

## STUDIES OF MANAGEMENT OF DEMENTIA

Scientists are now focusing on Alzheimer's disease, multi-infarct disease, and stroke. In time, we will learn to prevent or treat each disease. In the interim, the good news is what we have learned about caring for people with dementing illnesses. Much can be done to make life easier for the impaired person and his family. This book is one step in disseminating our growing understanding of ways to improve the quality of life in the presence of illness.

APPENDIXES

# 1. FURTHER READING

This reading list combines materials written primarily for the layman (marked with an *) and those written primarily for the professional. It is meant not to be a complete bibliography, but rather to get you started.

Bartol, M. 1979. Nonverbal Communication in Patients with Alzheimer's Disease. *Journal of Gerontological Nursing* 54 (July–August):21–31. [Although written for the professional, this may be helpful to families as well.]

Bergmann, K.; Foster, E. M.; Justice, A. W.; and Matthews, V. 1978. Management of the Demented Elderly Patient in the Community. *British Journal of Psychiatry* 132:441–49. [Demonstrates that family support allows patients to remain at home.]

Berkman, B. 1978. Mental Health and the Aging: A Review of Literature for Clinical Social Workers. *Clinical Social Work Journal* 6:230–45.

Brody, E. M. 1967. Aging Is a Family Affair, *Public Welfare* 25:129–40.

*———, 1977. *Long-Term Care of Older People*. New York: Human Sciences Press. [This is written for the professional but includes an excellent chapter for families.]

Brody, E. M., and Stark, G. 1966. Institutionalization of the Elderly: A Family Crisis. *Family Process* 5:76–90.

Brody, S.; Poulshock, S. W.; and Masciocci, C. F. 1978. The Family Care Unit: A Major Consideration in the Long Term Support System. *Gerontologist* 18:556–61.

Burnside, I. 1978. *Working with the Elderly: Group Processes and Techniques*. North Scituate, Mass.: Duxbury Press.

Burnside, I., ed. 1976. *Nursing and the Aged*. New York: McGraw-Hill.

Butler, R. N. 1979. Aging: Research Leads and Needs. *Forum on Medicine*, pp. 716–25. [Technical but readable review of where we stand.]

*Buter, R. N., and Lewis, M. I. 1976. *Sex after Sixty*. New York: Harper & Row.

Butler, R. N., and Lewis, M. I., eds. 1977. *Aging and Mental Health*. St. Louis: C. V. Mosby Co. [This general text is clearly written.]

*Carey, J. R. 1978. *How to Create Interiors for the Disabled*. New York: Pantheon Books. [Information applicable to the physically disabled but with clear illustrations to help you make modifications to your home for the impaired person. Remember that people with dementia may not be able to learn to use new equipment.]

Eisdorfer, C., and Friedel, R. 1977. *Cognitive and Emotional Disturbances in the Elderly*. Chicago: Year Book Medical Publishers.

Folstein, M. F., and McHugh, P. R. 1976. Phenomenological Approach to the Treatment of "Organic" Psychiatric Syndromes. In *The Therapists Handbook,* ed. B. Wolman, pp. 279–86. New York: Van Nostrand.

Freed, A. O. 1975. The Family Agency and Kinship System of the Elderly. *Social Casework* 56:579–86.

Gruenberg, E. 1978. Epidemiology of Senile Dementia. In *Advances in Neurology,* vol. 19, ed. B. Schoenberg, pp. 437–55, New York: Raven Press.

Gulevich, G. 1977. Psychopharmacological Treatment of the Aged. In *Psychopharmacology: From Theory to Practice*, ed. J. D. Barchas, P. A. Berger, R. D. Ciaranello, and G. R. Elliott, pp. 448–65. New York: Oxford.

*Hale, G., ed. 1979. *The Source Book for the Disabled*. New York: Paddington Press.

Herr, J., and Weakland, J. H. 1979. *Counseling Elders and Their Families*. New York: Springer Publishing Co.

*Jury, M., and Jury, D. 1976. *Gramp*. New York: Grossman Publishers. [A moving pictorial account of a man with a dementing illness who ages and dies at home.]

Kane, R., and Kane, R. 1980. Alternatives to the Institutional Care of the Elderly. *Gerontologist* 20:249–59.

Katzman, R. 1976. The Prevalence and Malignancy of Alzheimer's Disease, a Major Killer. *Archives of Neurology* 31:17–18.

Katzman, R.; Terry, R. D.; and Bick, K. L., eds. 1978. *Alzheimer's Disease: Senile Dementia and Related Disorders, Aging*, vol. 7. New York: Raven Press. [Excellent compilation of work done up to that time.]

*Kubler-Ross, E. 1970. *On Death and Dying*. New York: Macmillan.

Larsson, T.; Sjögren, T.; and Jacobson, G. 1963. Senile Dementia: A Clinical, Sociomedical and Genetic Study. *Acta Psychiatrica Scandinavica* (suppl. 167) 39:1–259.

LaVorgna, D. 1979. Group Treatment for Wives of Patients with Alzheimer's Disease. *Social Work in Health Care* 5:219–21.

Lawton, M. P. 1978. Institutions and Alternatives for Older People. *Health and Social Work* 3:108–34.

Lezak, M. 1978. Living with the Characterologically Altered Brain Injured Patient. *Journal of Clinical Psychiatry* 39:592–98. [Discusses problems families face.]

Lowy, L. 1979. *Social Work with the Aging*. New York: Harper & Row.

*McDowell, F. H., ed. 1980. *Managing the Person with Intellectual Loss (Dementia or Alzheimer's Disease) at Home*. White Plains, N.Y.: Burke Rehabilitation Center.

McHugh, P. R. 1979. Dementia. In *Textbook of Medicine*, 15th ed., ed. W. McDermott and J. B. Wyngaarden, pp. 660–61. Philadelphia: Saunders.

McHugh, P. R., and Folstein, M. F. 1979. Psychopathology of

Dementia: Implications for Neuropathology. In *Congenital and Acquired Cognitive Disorders*, ed. R. Katzman, pp. 17–30. New York: Raven Press.

*Nudel, A. 1979. *For the Woman over Fifty*. New York: Avon [Not about dementia, but full of resources and ideas for the midlife woman.]

*Otten, J., and Shelley, F. D. 1976. *When Your Parents Grow Old*. New York: Funk & Wagnalls. [Full of information and resources about aging in general.]

Parker, P., and Dietz, L. 1980. *Nursing at Home*. New York: Crown.

Pitt, B. 1975. *Psychogeriatrics*. Edinburgh: Churchill Livingstone.

Rabins, P. 1981. The Prevalence of Reversible Dementia in a Psychiatric Hospital, *Hospital and Community Psychiatry* 32:490–92.

Rathbone-McCuon, E., and Elliott, M. 1976. Geriatric Day Care in Theory and Practice. *Social Work in Health Care* 2:153–70.

Shanas, E. 1979. The Family as Social Support System in Old Age. *Gerontologist* 19:169–74.

Silverstone, B., and Miller, S. 1980. Isolation in the Aged: Individual Dynamics, Community and Family Involvement. *Journal of Geriatric Psychiatry* 13:27–47.

Sjögren, T.; Sjögren, H.; and Lindgren, A. G. H. 1952. "Clinical Analysis of Morbus Alzheimer and Morbus Pick." *Acta Psychiatrica et Neurologica Scandinavica* (suppl.) 82:1–152.

Strow, C., and Mackreth, R. 1977. Family Group Meetings: Strengthening a Partnership. *Journal of Gerontological Nursing* 3:30–35.

*Weinberg, J. 1974. What Do I Say to My Mother When I Have Nothing to Say. *Geriatrics* 29:155–59.

Wells, C. E., ed. 1977. *Dementia*. 2nd ed. Philadelphia: Davis.

Wolstenholme, G. E. W., and O'Connor, M. 1970. *Alzheimer's Disease and Related Disorders*. London: Churchill.

## Government Publications

Many of the publications listed below include names of voluntary organizations, other publications, or resources of value to concerned individuals. Specific inquiries concerning programs on the dementias may also be directed to the NINCDS Office of Scientific and Health

Reports, Bldg. 31, Room 8A–06, National Institutes of Health, Bethesda, MD 20205 (NIH), or to the Information Office, National Institute on Aging, Bldg. 31, Room 5C–36, National Institutes of Health, Bethesda, MD 20205 (NIA). Single copies of most publications are free.

*Alzheimer's Disease: A Scientific Guide for Health Practitioners.* NIH #81-2251.

*Alzheimer's Disease Q & A* NIH #80-1646.

*Aphasia: Hope through Research.* NIH #80-391.

*The Dementias: Hope through Research.* NIA #81-2252. [Excellent review of research, written for the layman.]

*Handle Yourself with Care,* Administration on Aging, Washington, D.C. 20201. [Safety tips.]

*Huntington's Disease: Hope through Research.* NIH #80-49.

*Multiple Sclerosis: Hope through Research.* NIH #79-75.

*Parkinson's Disease: Hope through Research.* NIH #76-139.

*Voluntary Health Agencies Working to Combat Neurological and Communicative Disorders.* NIH #81-74.

*What You Should Know about Stroke and Stroke Prevention.* NIH #79-1909.

You can get the tax forms and publications referred to in this book by writing to the IRS Forms Distribution Center listed in your Form 1040 or 1040A instructions. Or, you can call the tax information number in the phonebook listed under "United States Government, Internal Revenue Service."

Your local Social Security office can give you booklets explaining Social Security, Supplemental Security Income, and Medicare.

## 2. ORGANIZATIONS

Administration on Aging, 330 Independence Ave., S.W., Washington, DC 20201

Alexander Graham Bell Association for the Deaf, 2317 Volta Place, Washington, DC 20007

Alzheimer's Disease and Related Disorders Association, Inc., 360 N. Michigan Ave., Chicago, IL 60601 (national office; local chapter addresses are available upon request)

American Association of Homes for the Aging, 1050 17th St., N.W., Washington, DC 20036

American Association of Retired Persons, 1909 K. St., N.W., Washington, DC 20006

American Cancer Society, 219 East 42nd St., New York, NY 10021

American Diabetes Association, 18 East 48th St., New York, NY 10017

American Foundation for the Blind, 15 West 16th St., New York, NY 10011

American Geriatrics Society, 10 Columbus Circle, New York, NY 10019

American Heart Association, 44 East 23rd St., New York, NY 10010

American Lung Association, 1740 Broadway, New York, NY 10019

American Nurses Association, Inc., 10 Columbus Circle, New York, NY 10019

American Nursing Home Association (American Health Care Association), 1025 Connecticut Ave., N.W., Washington, DC 20036

American Occupational Therapy Association, 1383 Picard Drive, Rockville, MD 20850

American Parkinson's Disease Association, Rm 602, 47 E. 50th St., New York, NY 10022

American Physical Therapy Association, 1740 Broadway, New York, NY 10019

American Psychological Association, Division of Adult Development and Aging, 1200 17th St., N.W., Washington, DC 20036

Arthritis Foundation, 1212 Avenue of the Americas, New York, NY 10036

Association of Rehabilitation Facilities, 5530 Wisconsin Ave., N.W., Washington, DC 20015 (For information about rehabilitation centers across the country serving older people.)

Cancer Care, One Park Ave., New York, NY 10016

Family Service Association of America, 44 East 23rd St., New York, NY 10010

Gerontological Society, 1 Dupont Circle, N.W., Washington, DC 20036 (Professional association for studies of aging in the biological sciences, clinical medicine, psychological and social sciences, and social research, planning, and practice.)

Gray Panthers, 3700 Chestnut St., Philadelphia, PA 19104 (Activist organization of old and young people concerned with issues of aging.)

National Association for Mental Health, 1800 North Kent St., Arlington, VA 22209

National Association for the Deaf, 814 Thayer Ave., Silver Spring, MD 20910

National Association for Visually Handicapped, 305 East 24th St., New York, NY 10010

National Association of Hearing and Speech Agencies, 814 Thayer Ave., Silver Spring, MD 20910

National Association of Social Workers, 1425 H St., N.W., Suite 600, Washington, DC 20005

National Council for Homemakers, Home Health Aide Services, 1790 Broadway, New York, NY 10019

National Council of Health Care Services, 407 N St., S.W., Washington, DC 20024

National Council of Senior Citizens, 1511 K St., N.W., Washington, DC 20005

National Council on the Aging, 600 Maryland Ave., S.W., Washington, DC 20024 (Information, services, and research on aging. Publications on day care and senior centers, retirement housing.)

National Federation of Licensed Practical Nurses, 250 W. 57th St., New York, NY 10001

National Institute of Neurological and Communicative Disorders and Stroke, Office of Scientific and Health Reports, Bldg. 31, Room 8A-06, National Institutes of Health, Bethesda, MD 20205

National Institute on Aging, Information Office, Bldg. 31, Room 5C-36, National Institutes of Health, Bethesda, MD 20205

National Society for the Prevention of Blindness, Inc., 79 Madison Ave., New York, NY 10016

## 3. WHERE TO BUY OR RENT SUPPLIES

Incontinence supplies, eating aids, bathroom aids, wheelchairs, geriatric chairs, etc.:

Sears, Roebuck and Co. (ask for their home health care catalog)
Medical supply houses, listed in the yellow pages of telephone directories.

Diapers:
> Adult diaper services, listed in the yellow pages of telephone directories under "Diaper Services."

Medicare publishes a list of the supplies and rentals they cover. The medical supply house can also tell you which items are covered by your insurance.

Information about Medic Alert may be available through local pharmacies or you can write to Medic Alert, Turlock, CA 95380.

## 4. U.S. STATE AND PROTECTORATE AGENCIES

These agencies are designated to administer programs that serve the elderly.

ALABAMA

Commission on Aging, 740 Madison Ave., Montgomery 36104

ALASKA

Department of Health and Social Services, Pouch H, Juneau 99811
Office on Aging, Department of Health and Social Services, Pouch H, Juneau 99811

ARIZONA

Department of Economic Security, 1717 West Jefferson, Phoenix 85007
Bureau on Aging, Department of Economic Security, P.O. Box 6123, Phoenix 85004

ARKANSAS

Department of Human Services, 406 National Old Lind Bldg., Little Rock 72201
Office on Aging and Adult Services, Department of Human Services, 7107 West 12th St., P.O. Box 2179, Little Rock, 72203

CALIFORNIA

Health and Welfare Agency, 926 J St., Room 917, Sacramento 95814

Department of Aging, Health and Welfare Agency, 918 J St., Sacramento 95814

COLORADO

Department of Social Services, 1575 Sherman St., Denver 80203
Division of Services for the Aging, Department of Social Services, 1575 Sherman St., Denver 80203

CONNECTICUT

Department on Aging, 90 Washington St., Room 312, Hartford 06115

DELAWARE

Department of Health and Social Services, Delaware State Hospital, 3rd floor Administration Bldg., New Castle 19720
Division of Aging, Department of Health and Social Services, New Castle 19720

DISTRICT OF COLUMBIA

Office of Aging, Office of the Mayor, 1012 14th St., N.W., Suite 1106, Washington, DC 20005

FLORIDA

Department of Health and Rehabilitation Services, 1323 Winewood Blvd., Tallahassee 32301
Program Office of Aging and Adult Services, Department of Health and Rehabilitation Services, 1323 Winewood Blvd., Tallahassee 32301

GEORGIA

Department of Human Resources, 618 Ponce de Leon Ave., N.E., Atlanta 30308
Office of Aging, Department of Human Resources, 618 Ponce de Leon Ave., N.E., Atlanta 30308

GUAM

Department of Public Health and Social Services, Government of Guam, P.O. Box 2816, Agana 96910

Office of Aging, Social Service Administration, Government of Guam, P.O. Box 2816, Agana 96910

HAWAII

Executive Office on Aging, Office of the Governor, State of Hawaii, 1149 Bethel St., Room 307, Honolulu 96813

IDAHO

Idaho Office on Aging, Statehouse, Boise 83720

ILLINOIS

Department on Aging, 2401 West Jefferson, Springfield 62706

INDIANA

Commission on Aging and Aged, Graphic Arts Bldg., 215 North Senate Ave., Indianapolis 46202

IOWA

Commission on Aging, 415 West 10th St., Jewett Bldg., Des Moines 50319

KANSAS

Department of Aging, Biddle Bldg., 2700 West 6th St., Topeka 66606

KENTUCKY

Department for Human Resources, Capital Annex, Room 201, Frankfort 40601

Center for Aging and Community Development, Department for Human Resources, 403 Wapping St., Frankfort 40601

LOUISIANA

Health and Human Resources Administration, P.O. Box 44215, Capitol Station, Baton Rouge 70804

Bureau of Aging Services, Division of Human Resources, Health and Human Resources Administration, P.O. Box 44282, Capitol Station, Baton Rouge 70804

MAINE

Department of Human Services, State House, Augusta 04333

Bureau of Maine's Elderly, Community Services Unit, Department of Human Services, State House, Augusta 04333

MARYLAND

Office on Aging, State Office Bldg., 301 West Preston St., Baltimore 21201

MASSACHUSETTS

Department of Elder Affairs, 110 Tremont St., Boston 02108

MICHIGAN

Office of Services to the Aging, 300 East Michigan, P.O. Box 30026, Lansing 48909

MINNESOTA

Governor's Citizens Council on Aging, Suite 204 Metro Square Bldg., 7th and Robert Sts., St. Paul 55101

MISSISSIPPI

Council on Aging, P.O. Box 5136, Fondren Station, 510 George St., Jackson 39216

MISSOURI

Department of Social Services, Broadway State Office Bldg., P.O. Box 570, Jefferson City 65101
Office of Aging, Division of Special Services, Department of Social Services, Broadway State Office Bldg., P.O. Box 570, Jefferson City 65101

MONTANA

Department of Social and Rehabilitation Services, P.O. Box 1723, Helena 58601
Aging Services Bureau, Department of Social and Rehabilitation Services, P.O. Box 1723, Helena 59601

NEBRASKA

Commission on Aging, State House Station 94784, P.O. Box 95044, Lincoln 68509

Nevada

Department of Human Resources, 505 East King St., Room 600, Carson City 89710

Division for Aging Services, Department of Human Resources, 505 East King St., Room 600, Carson City 89710

New Hampshire

Council on Aging, P.O. Box 786, 14 Depot St., Concord 03301

New Jersey

Division on Aging, Department of Community Affairs, P.O. Box 2768, 363 West State St., Trenton 08625

New Mexico

Commission on Aging, 408 Galisteo-Villagra Bldg., Santa Fe 87503

New York

Office for the Aging, Agency Bldg. 2, Empire State Plaza, Albany 12223

New York City Field Office FYI

2 World Trade Center, Room 5036, New York 10047

North Carolina

Department of Human Resources, Albermarle Bldg., Raleigh 27603

North Carolina Division for Aging, Department of Human Resources, 213 Hillsborough St., Raleigh 27603

North Dakota

Social Services Board of North Dakota, State Capitol Bldg., Bismarck 58505

Aging Services, Social Services Board of North Dakota, State Capitol Bldg., Bismarck 58505

Ohio

Commission on Aging, 50 West Broad St., Columbus 43216

Oklahoma

Department of Institutions, Social and Rehabilitative Services, P.O. Box 25352, Oklahoma City 73125

Special Unit on Aging, Department of Institutions, Social and Rehabilitative Services, P.O. Box 25352, Oklahoma City 73125

OREGON

Human Resources Department, 315 Public Service Bldg., Salem 97310

Office of Elderly Affairs, Human Resources Department, 772 Commercial St., S.E., Salem 97310

PENNSYLVANIA

Department of Public Welfare, Health and Welfare Bldg., Harrisburg 17120

Office for the Aging, Department of Public Welfare, Health and Welfare Bldg., Rm. 540, P.O. Box 2675, 7th & Forster St., Harrisburg 17120

PUERTO RICO

Department of Social Services, P.O. Box 11398, Santurce 00910

Gericulture Commission, Department of Social Services, P.O. Box 11398, Santurce 00910

RHODE ISLAND

Department of Community Affairs, 150 Washington Ct., Providence 02903

Division on Aging, Department of Community Affairs, 150 Washington Ct., Providence 02903

SAMOA

Territorial Administration on Aging, Government of American Samoa, Pago Pago, American Samoa 96799

SOUTH CAROLINA

Commission on Aging, 915 Main St., Columbia 29201

SOUTH DAKOTA

Department of Social Services, State Office Bldg., Illinois St., Pierre 57501

Office on Aging, Department of Social Services, State Office Bldg., Illinois St., Pierre 57501

TENNESSEE

Commission on Aging, Room 102 S & P Bldg., 306 Gay St., Nashville 37201

TEXAS

Governor's Committee on Aging, Executive Office Bldg., 411 W. 13th St. Floors 4 & 5, Austin 78703

TRUST TERRITORY OF THE PACIFIC

Office of Aging, Community Development Division, Government of the Trust Territory of the Pacific Islands, Saipan, Mariana Islands 96950

UTAH

Department of Social Services, State Capitol Bldg., Room 221, Salt Lake City 84102

Division of Aging, Department of Social Services, 150 West North Temple, Salt Lake City 84102

VERMONT

Agency of Human Services, 79 River St., Montpelier 05602

Office on Aging, Agency of Human Services, 81 River St. (Heritage 1), Montpelier 05602

VIRGINIA

Office on Aging, 830 East Main St., Suite 950, Richmond 23219

VIRGIN ISLANDS

Commission on Aging, P.O. Box 539, Charlotte Amalie, St. Thomas 00801

WASHINGTON

Department of Social and Health Services, P.O. Box 1788, M.S. 45–2, Olympia 98504

Office on Aging, Department of Social and Health Services, P.O. Box 1788, M.S. 45–2, Olympia 98504

WEST VIRGINIA

Commission on Aging, State Capitol, Charleston 25305

WISCONSIN

Department of Health and Social Services, State Office Bldg., Room 700, 1 West Wilson St., Madison 53702

Division on Aging, Department of Health and Social Services, 1 West Wilson St., Room 686, Madison 53702

WYOMING

Department of Health and Social Services, Division of Public Assistance, New State Office Bldg. West, Room 380, Cheyenne 82002

Aging Services, Department of Health and Social Services, Division of Public Assistance and Social Services, New State Office Bldg. West, Room 288, Cheyenne 82002

## 5. RIGHTS OF HOSPITAL AND NURSING HOME PATIENTS

Most state departments of health publish bills of rights for patients in hospitals and nursing homes, and you can obtain copies from your own state health department. You and your parent(s) should be familiar with these rights. In general, they will follow those outlined here (reprinted from Jane Otten and Florence D. Shelley, *When Your Parents Grow Old* [New York: Funk and Wagnalls, 1976, by permission of Harper & Row, Publishers, Inc.])

## Hospital Patients Bill of Rights

The patient should have the right:
1. To considerate and respectful care.
2. To receive, upon request, the name of the physician responsible for coordinating his care.
3. To know the name and function of any person providing health-care services for the patient.
4. To obtain from his physician complete current information concerning his diagnosis, treatment, and prognosis in terms the patient can reasonably be expected to understand. When it is not medically advisable to give such information to the patient, the information shall be made available to an appropriate person in his behalf.

5. To receive from his physician information necessary to give informed consent prior to the start of any procedure or treatment or both, and which, except for those emergency situations not requiring informed consent, shall include as a minimum the specific procedure or treatment or both, the medically significant risks involved, and the probable duration of incapacitation, if any. The patient shall be advised of medically significant alternatives for care or treatment, if any.

6. To refuse treatment to the extent permitted by law and to be informed of the medical consequences of his action.

7. To privacy to the extent consistent with providing adequate medical care to the patient. This shall not preclude discreet discussion of a patient's case or examination of a patient by appropriate health-care personnel.

8. To privacy and confidentiality of all records pertaining to the patient's treatment, except as otherwise provided by law or third-party-payment contract.

9. To a response by the hospital, in a reasonable manner, to the patient's request for services customarily rendered by the hospital consistent with the patient's treatment.

10. To be informed by his physician or a delegate of the physician of the patient's continuing health-care requirements following discharge; and to be informed by the hospital, before transferral to another facility, of the need for, and alternatives to, such a transfer.

11. To know the identity, upon request, of other health-care and educational institutions that the hospital has authorized to participate in his treatment.

12. To refuse to participate in research or human experimentation without his consent.

13. To examine and receive an explanation of his bill, regardless of source of payment.

14. To know the hospital rules and regulations that apply to his conduct as a patient.

15. To treatment without discrimination as to race, color, religion, sex, national origin, or source of payment.

# Nursing Home Patients Bill of Rights

The nursing home must assure that each patient:

1. Is fully informed, as evidenced by the patient's written acknowledgment, prior to or at the time of admission, and during stay, of these rights and of all rules and regulations governing patient conduct and responsibilities.

2. Is fully informed, prior to or at the time of admission, and during stay, of services available in the facility, and of related charges, including any charges for services not covered by sources of third-party payments or not covered by the facility's per-diem rate.

3. Is fully informed, by a physician, of his medical condition unless medically contraindicated (as documented, by a physician, in his medical record), and is afforded the opportunity to participate in experimental research.

4. Is transferred or discharged only for medical reasons, or for his welfare or that of other patients, or for nonpayment of his stay (except as prohibited by sources of third-party payment), and is given reasonable advance notice to ensure orderly transfer or discharge, and such actions are documented in his medical record.

5. Is encouraged and assisted, throughout his period of stay, to exercise his rights as a patient and as a citizen, and to this end may voice grievances and recommended changes in policies and services to facility staff and/or to outside representatives of his choice, free from restraint, interference, coercion, discrimination, or reprisal.

6. May manage his personal financial affairs, or is given at least a quarterly accounting of financial transactions made on his behalf should the facility accept his written delegation of this responsibility to the facility for any period of time in conformance with state law.

7. Is free from mental and physical abuse, and free from chemical and (except in emergencies) physical restraints, except as authorized in writing by a physician for a specified and limited period of time, or when necessary to protect the patient from injury to himself or to others.

8. Is assured confidential treatment of his personal and medical records, and may approve or refuse their release to any individual outside the facility, except in the case of his transfer to another health-care institution.

9. Is treated with consideration, respect, and full recognition of his dignity and individuality, including privacy in treatment and in care for his personal needs.

10. Is not required to perform services for the facility that are not included for therapeutic purposes in his plan of care.

11. May associate and communicate privately with persons of his choice, and send and receive his personal mail unopened, unless medically contraindicated.

12. May meet with and participate in activities of social, religious, and community groups at his discretion, unless medically contraindicated.

13. May retain and use his personal clothing and possessions as space permits, unless to do so would infringe upon rights of other patients, and unless medically contraindicated.

14. If married, is assured privacy for visits by his/her spouse; if both are in-patients in the facility, they are permitted to share a room, unless medically contraindicated.

# INDEX

# Index

# Index

# Index

Clergy, 229–30, 263, 307. *See also* Counseling

Clinging, 151–52. *See also* Demands of patient

Clock, 36; internal, 53–54, 140; and patient's inability to tell time, 53–54

Clothing, 95–96; as cause of sores or pain, 111; cost of, 277; in nursing home, 307; to prevent patient from undressing, 145–48; refusal to change, 64, 91–92. *See also* Dressing, helping the patient in; Incontinence

Clumsiness. *See* Coordination problems

Coffee, overuse of, 259–60

Colds, as cause of delirium, 109

Color discrimination, 118–20

Combativeness, 37–41, 167–68; following seizure, 123

Commode. *See* Toilet

Communication problems, 13, 14, 34, 35, 41–49, 102, 103, 111, 115, 119, 238, 309–12, 322–23, 325. *See also* Family

Community education. *See* Education

Complaints, 153–57; about nursing home, 311. *See also* Accusations; Advocacy; Criticism; Insults

Complete blood count (CBC), 21

Computerized axial tomogram (CAT scan), 22

Concealing illness, 11, 43, 129–30

Conflict in families. *See* Family

Confusion: following seizure, 123; at night, 140–44. *See also* specific behaviors

Consent form, 280

Conservatorship, 282

Constipation, 79, 86, 97, 103, 111, 114–15

Contact lenses, 84

Control. *See* Alcohol use/abuse; Incontinence; Independence; Roles

Convulsion. *See* Seizure

Cooking; with aluminum utensils, 333; as fire hazard, 75; learning, 208; if patient has stopped, 65; *See also* Meals

Coordination problems, 13, 49–53, 71, 95, 106–108; assessing, 24; in driving, 62; *See also* Dressing, helping the patient in; Eating; Falling; Vision

Cortical function testing, 23

Cosmetics. *See* Make-up, for patient

Coughing, 111

Counseling, 166, 236, 240, 246–247, 258–64; for children 272–73; for family, 219; for groups, 266; for patient, 32; sexual, 148

Creutzfeldt-Jacob disease, 333

Criticism, 39, 153–57, 213, 229. *See also* Accusations; Family

Crying, *See* Catastrophic reactions; Depression; Grief

Cushions, 113

Custodial care, 295

Daily care. *See* specific activities

Dancing, as exercise, 87

Dating, 251

Day care center: adult, 201–202; patient wandering away from, 131–140

Day hospital, 201

Deafness. *See* hearing problems

Death: care of patient in event of care giver's, 185–87; cause of, 125; decisions about, 84, 125–

362

# Index

# Index

# Index

Food. *See* Diet; Eating; Meals

Forgetfulness. *See* Memory aids; Memory problems

Foster care, 276, 290

Fracture. *See* Injury

Friedreich's ataxia, 321

Friends, 129, 256–57, 288; children's 224; drifting away of, 250, 254; finding, in volunteer groups, 264–265; help from, 195–96; importance of, for care giver, 233, 236, 240, 256–57; patient visiting with, 40, 89; when patient accuses or insults, 155, 178. *See also* Dating

Frustration: of family/care giver, 227–31; of patient, 164. *See also* Catastrophic reactions

Funding. *See* Resources, financial

Funeral, 127, 186–87

Furniture, 52, 74, 101, 107

Genetics, 335

Genitals: cleaning, 94; exposing, 145–48

Geri-chair, 139

Gesture. *See* Body language

Glasses. *See* Eyeglasses

Grab bars, 75, 94, 99, 194

Grief, 209, 223, 237–39, 258, 292, 312. *See also* Depression

Grooming, personal, 64, 91–92, 96–97

Guardianship, 282–83

Guilt, 178–79, 210, 233–36, 256, 258, 292, 312

Hair care, 96–97

Hallucination, 13, 111, 171–81, 325. *See also* Agnosia (failure to recognize things); Delusion; Sleep, patient's problems obtaining

Handicapped persons, 192, 244

Hand rails, 74, 107. *See also* Grab bars

Hardening of arteries. *See* Multiinfarct disease

Hazards, 71–77, 94, 131, 139, 140, 165; of driving, 60–63; fire, 140–43; of medications, 116–18; at night, 143; in nursing home, 302–308; of swimming pools, 138; of wandering, 131–33; when patient lives alone, 63–66

Headache, 110, 115, 123

Head injuries, 22, 108, 123, 320, 326–27

Health insurance. *See* Insurance

Hearing aid, paying for, 193

Hearing problems, 46, 120–21, 171–72; and driving, 60–61. *See also* Agnosia (failure to recognize things); Hallucination

Heart problems, 78, 87, 111, 331

Help: counseling as, 258–65; in emergencies, 183–85; finding additional, 15, 189–201; at home, 196–99. *See also* Family; Sitter

Helplessness, feelings of, 231–32. *See also* Independence

Hematoma, 320. *See also* Head injuries

Heredity, 335

Hiding: objects, 145, 171–81; important papers, 284–86. *See also* Catastrophic reactions

High blood pressure. *See* Hypertension

Hitting, 34–41, 124, 167–68; of patient by care giver, 260. *See also* Catastrophic reactions

Hoarding. *See* Hiding

# Index

# Index

# Index

# Index

# Index

# Index

# Index

# Index

# Improve Your Health
# With WARNER BOOKS

# For Every Kitchen

___THE ALLERGY COOKBOOK & FOOD-BUYING GUIDE
Pamela P. Nonken and                    (L37-901, $7.95, U.S.A.)
S. Roger Hirsch, M.D.                    (L37-902, $9.95, Canada)
Pamela Nonken, whose daughter is allergic to yeast, determined
to devise a workable diet that included bread products but ex-
cluded yeast . . . and one so delicious that all her family could
enjoy it too. She succeeded so well that Dr. Roger Hirsch, a
practicing allergist, asked her to expand her efforts and design
recipes that would exclude five other common allergens—corn,
soy, wheat, eggs, and milk.

___THE CAROB WAY TO HEALTH    (L37-302, $5.95, U.S.A.)
Frances Sheridan Goulart       (L37-315, $7.25, Canada)
If chocolate doesn't like you, try Mother Nature's perfect treat:
carob, the chocolate taste-alike that's everything you ever
dreamed about—and less. It's all here, from the wonderpod's
ancient history to its uses in cooking and herbal medicine—
dozens of delectable recipes for main dishes and accompani-
ments, frostings, fillings, sauces, beverages, and, of course,
candies and snacks.

___THE GOOD HEART DIET COOKBOOK
Ellen Stern & Jonathan Michaels    (L37-547, $6.95, U.S.A.)
Foreword by Siegfried J. Kra, M.D.  (L37-212, $8.50, Canada)
Who needs this book? All of you who . . . can't sit through a movie
without buttered popcorn, like your asparagus with hollandaise,
grab a burger and a soda for a quick bite, have hypertension, are
diabetic, have a high cholesterol count, have a family history of
heart disease, have arthritis, or are overweight.

Do you face a life of days that seem 36 hours long — tending someone who can no longer think and remember, someone who is slowly slipping out of being the person you love?

## Then THE 36-HOUR DAY is for you.

Nancy L. Mace and Peter V. Rabins, M.D. combine practical advice with specific examples in this comprehensive guide to the care of those in the early and middle stages of Alzheimer's disease and related illnesses. *The 36-Hour Day* covers the medical, legal, financial, and emotional aspects of caring for an impaired relative, including:

- Finding the right doctor, nurse, and/or social worker
- Avoiding hazards in the home related to meals, medicine, hygiene, exercise, and balance
- Getting outside help from friends, neighbors, lawyers
- Assessing financial obligations — potential expenses and resources
- Caring for yourself — taking time out for counseling, support groups, friendships
- Dealing with anger, embarrassment, depression, and fatigue
- Understanding medical research — studies of heredity, contributing diseases, nutrition, brain structures, drugs, and physical activity

32201

0

7 70993 00395

ISBN 0-446-32201-6

COVER PRINTED IN U.S.A.
1984 WARNER BOOKS